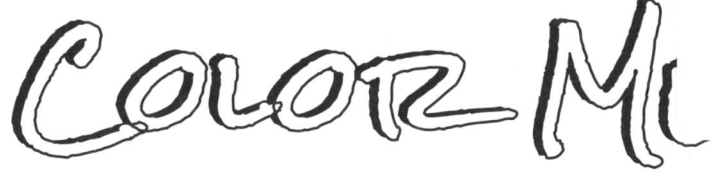 

31 Day Clean & Sober Coloring Journal

Day By Day Recovery Resources LLC

Day-By-Day.org

Copyright 2017 © All rights reserved.

ISBN 978-1-934569-46-7

LCCN 2017951688

Printed in PRC

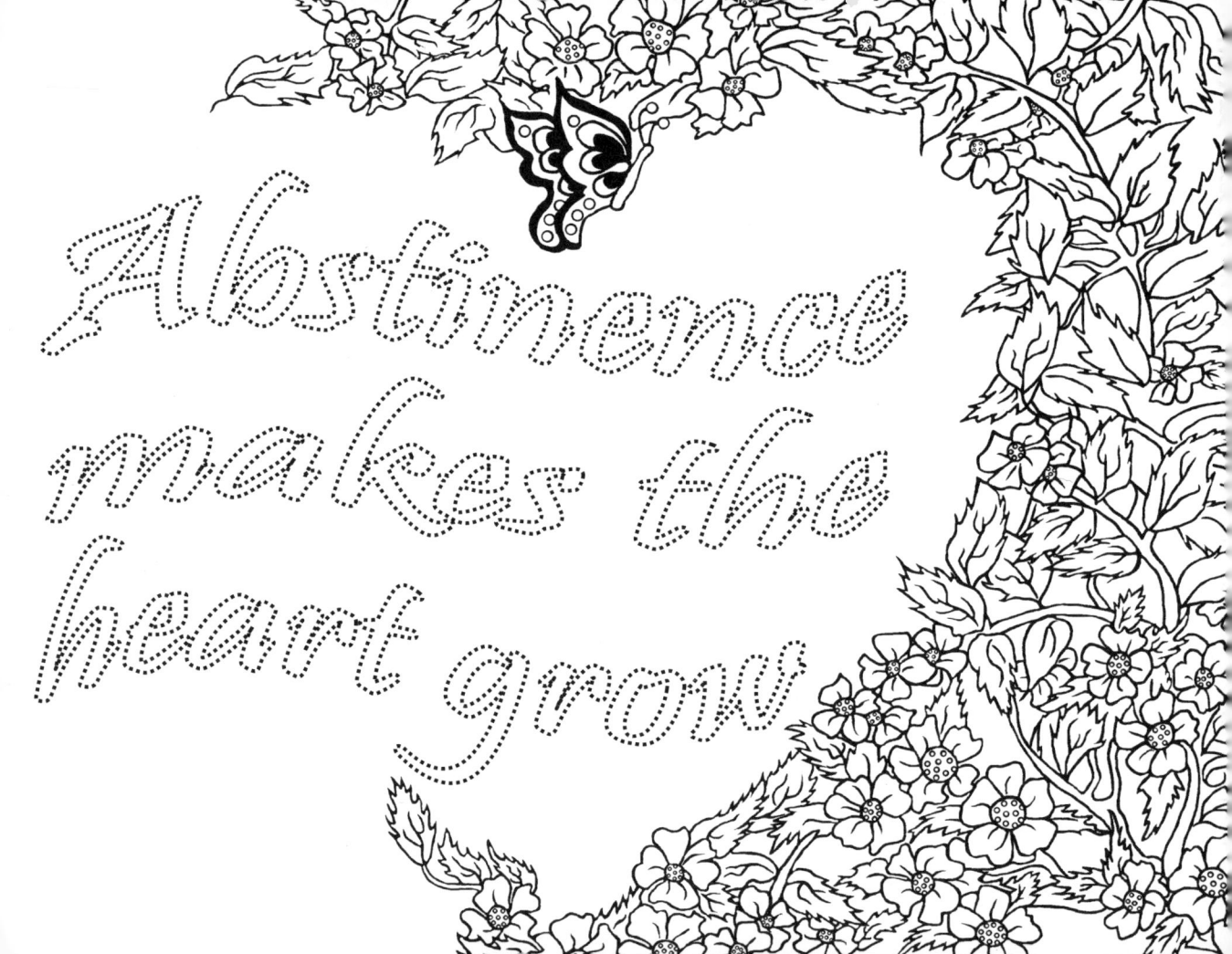

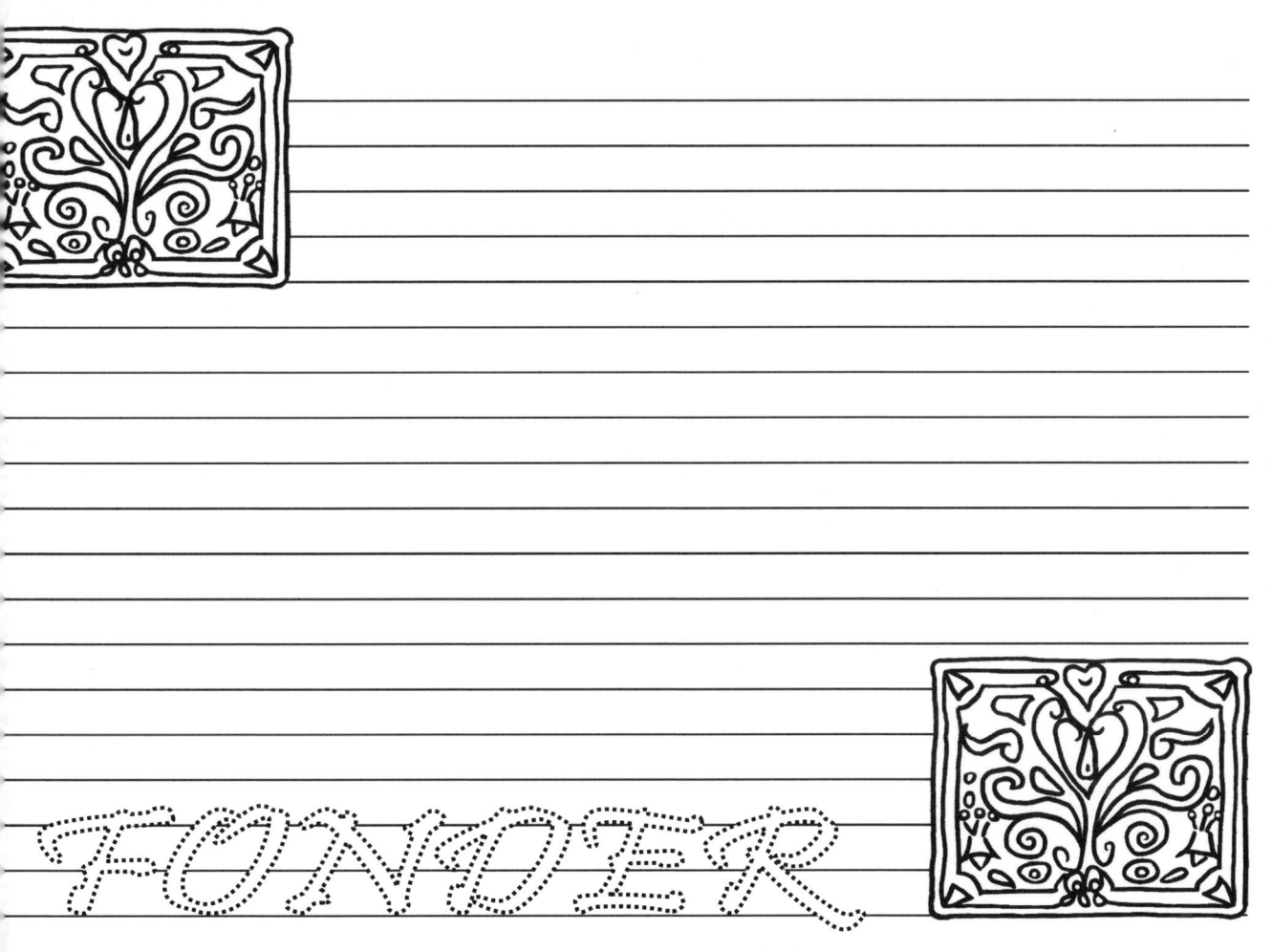

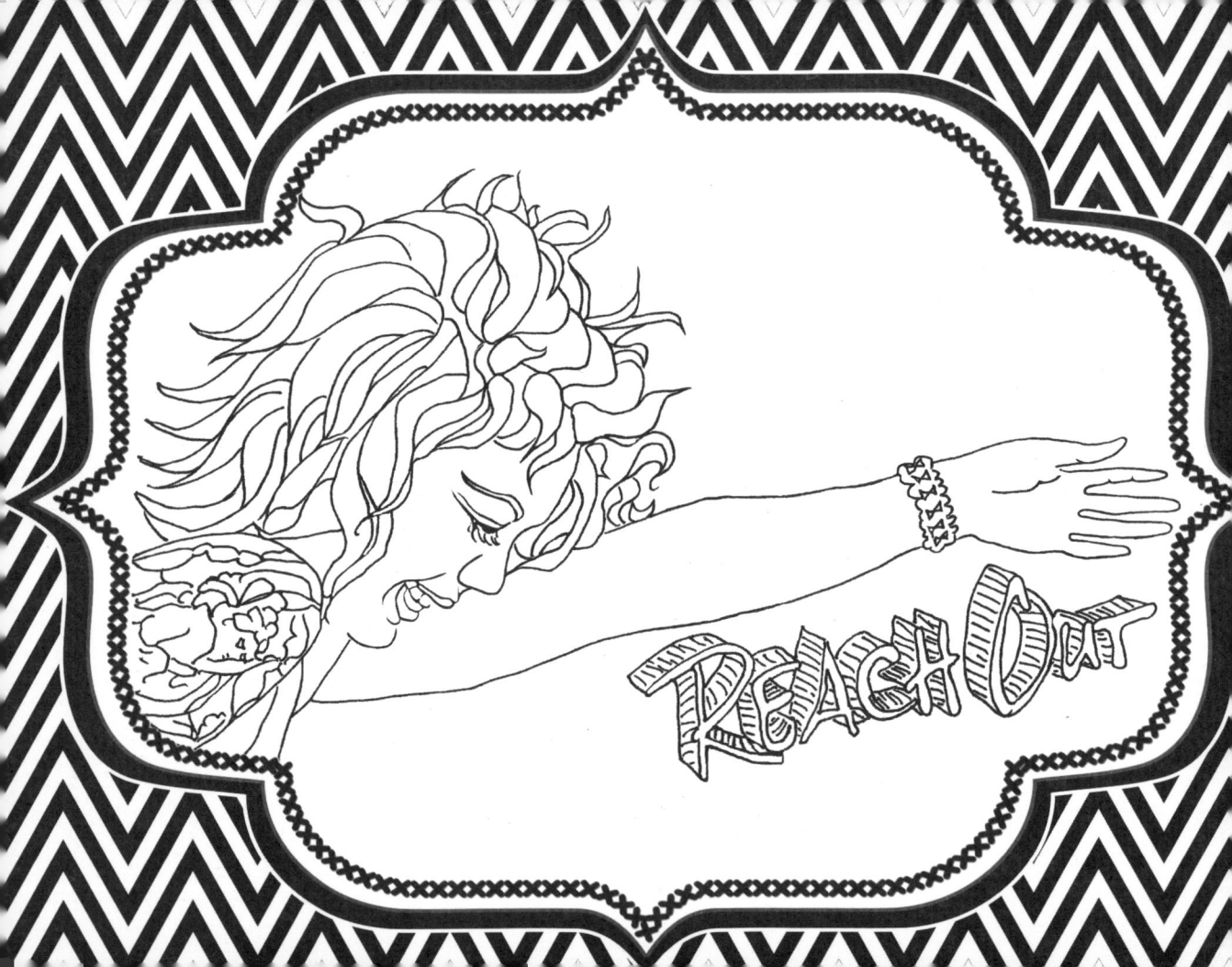

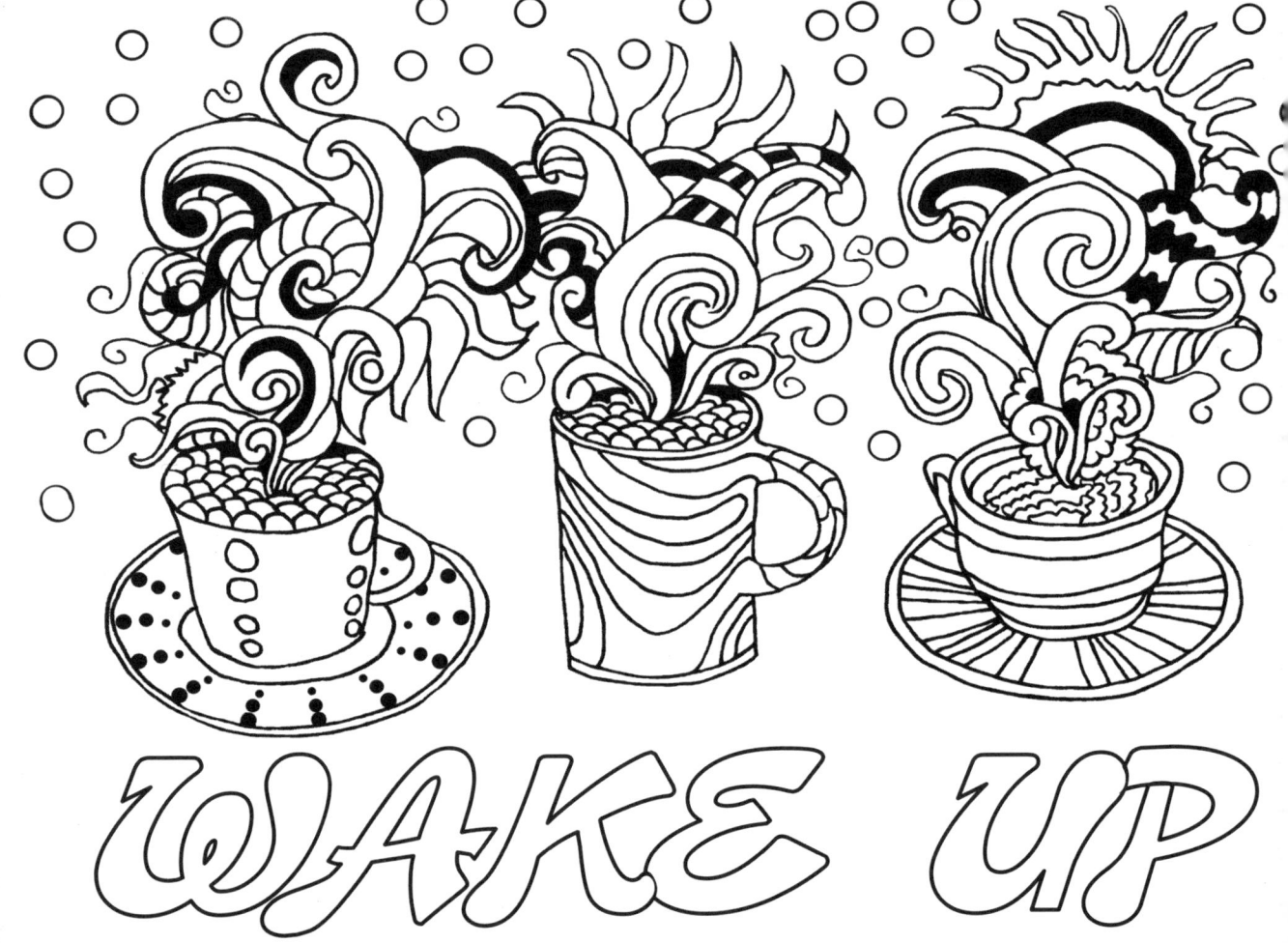

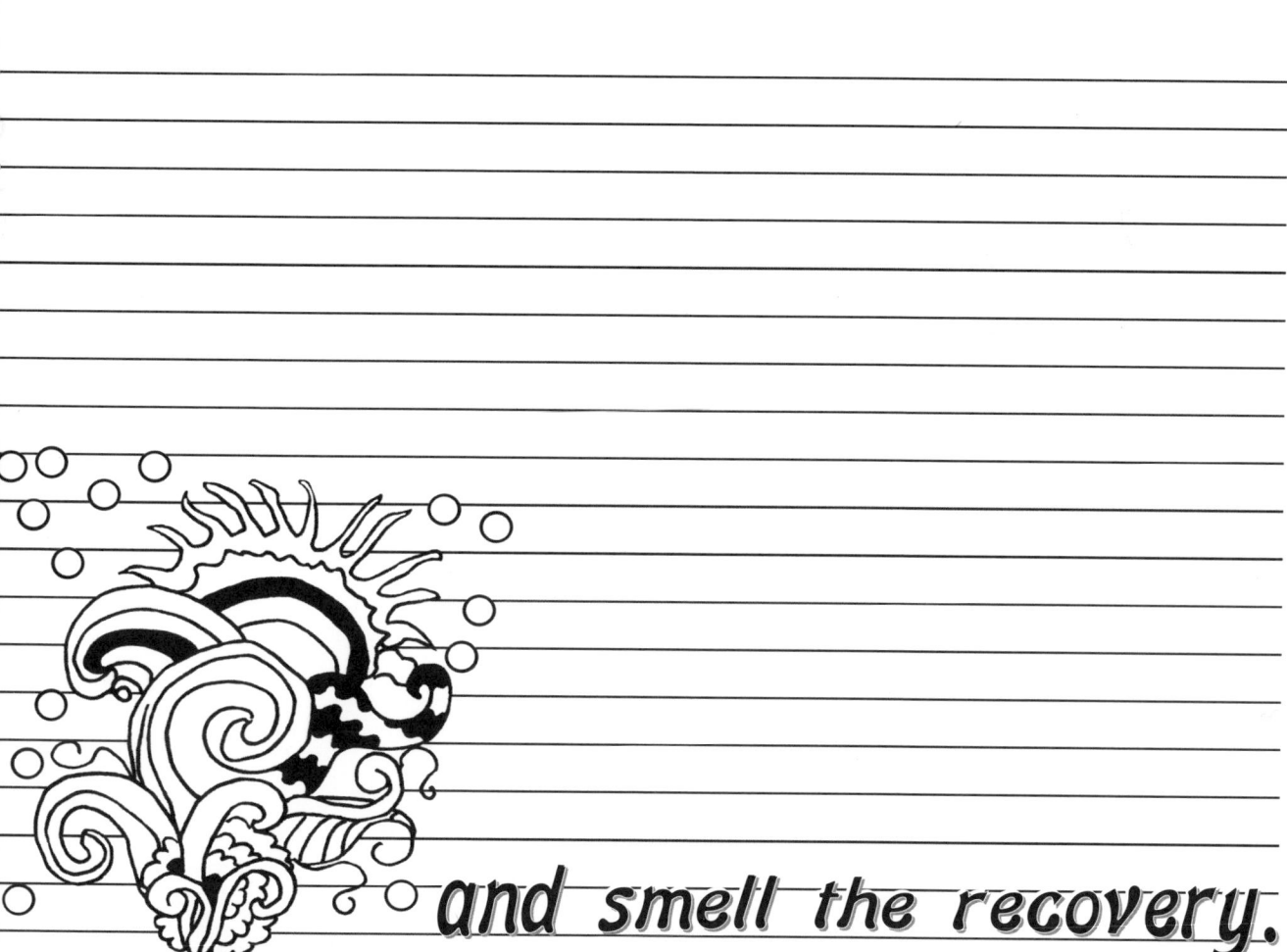

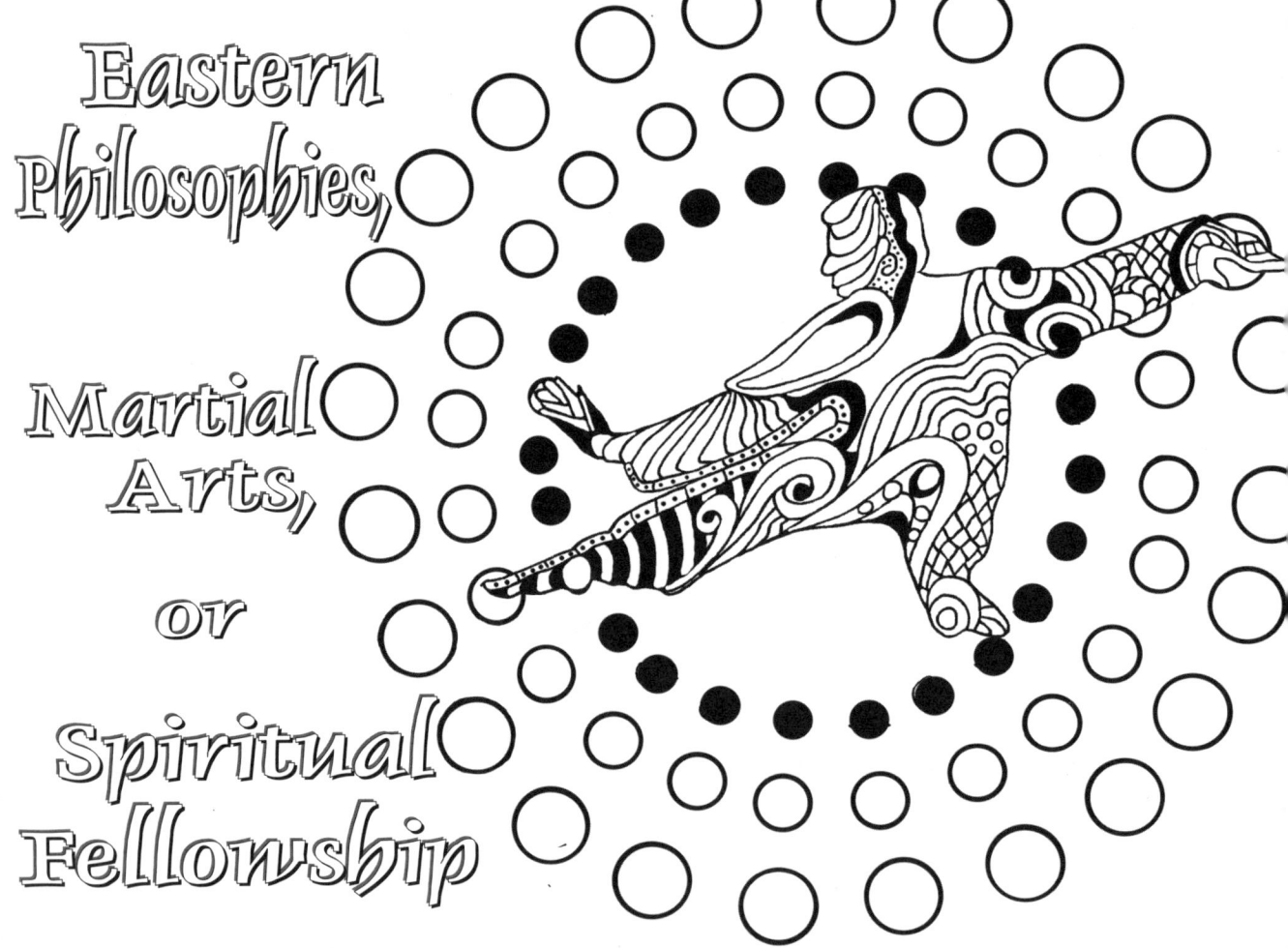

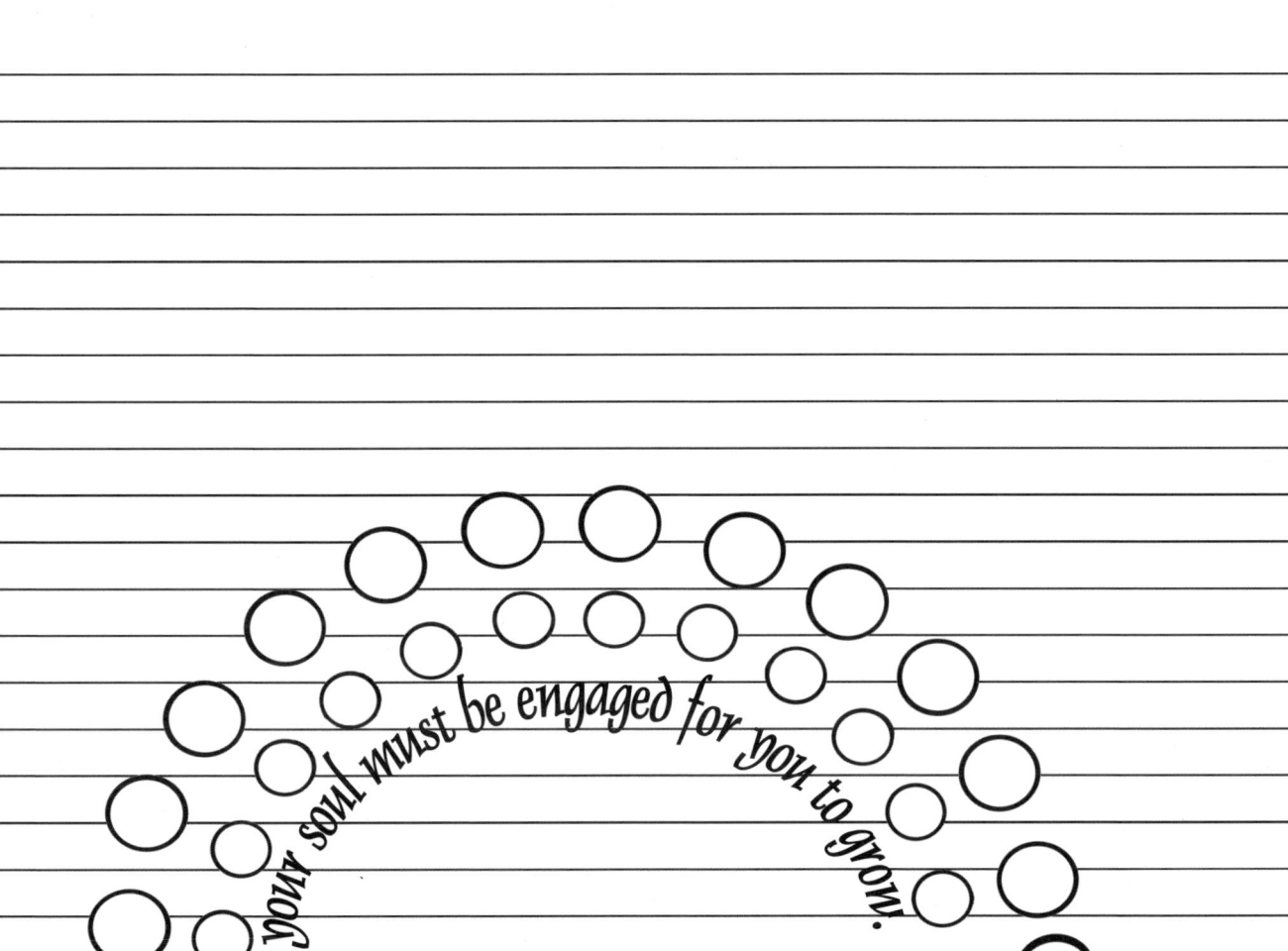

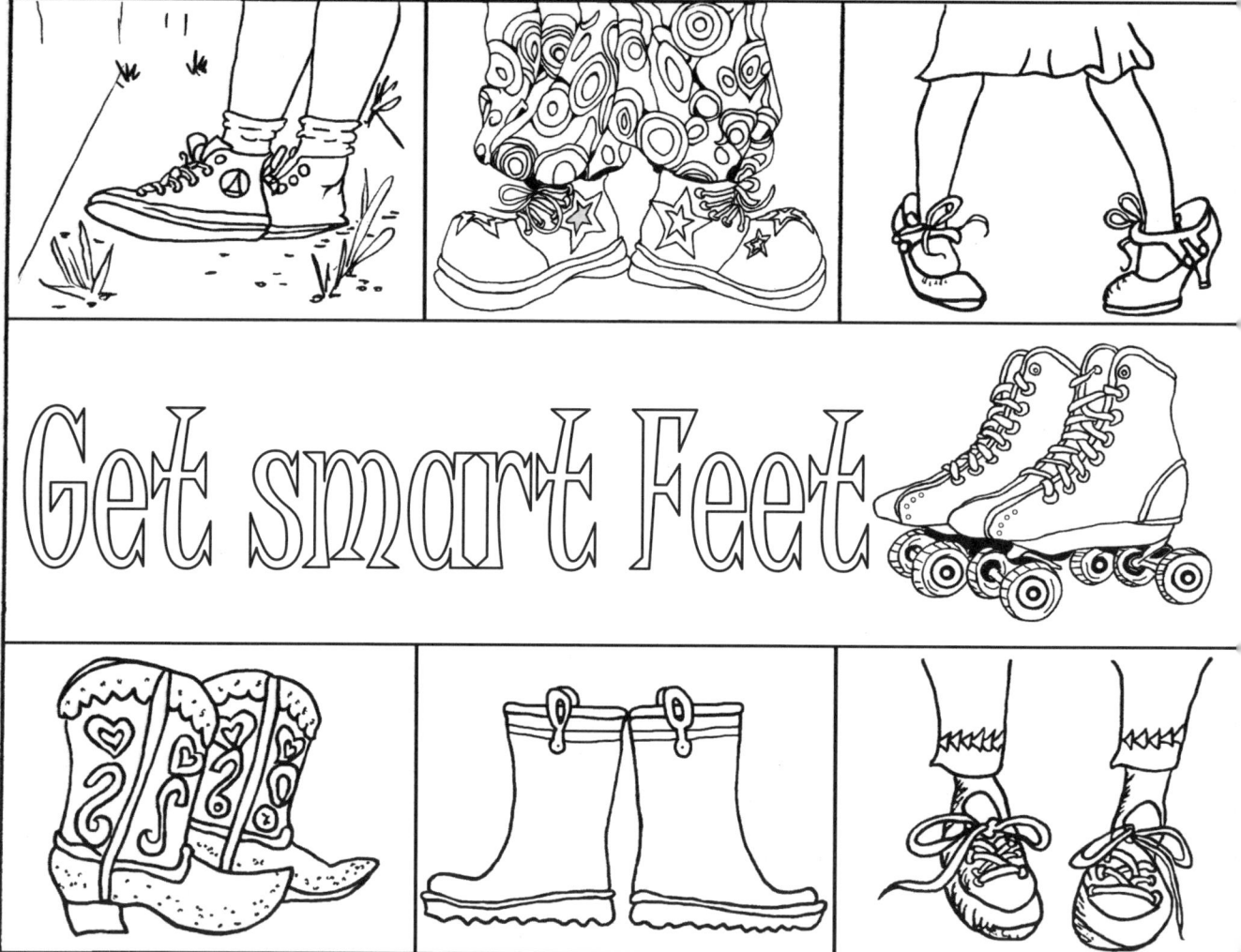

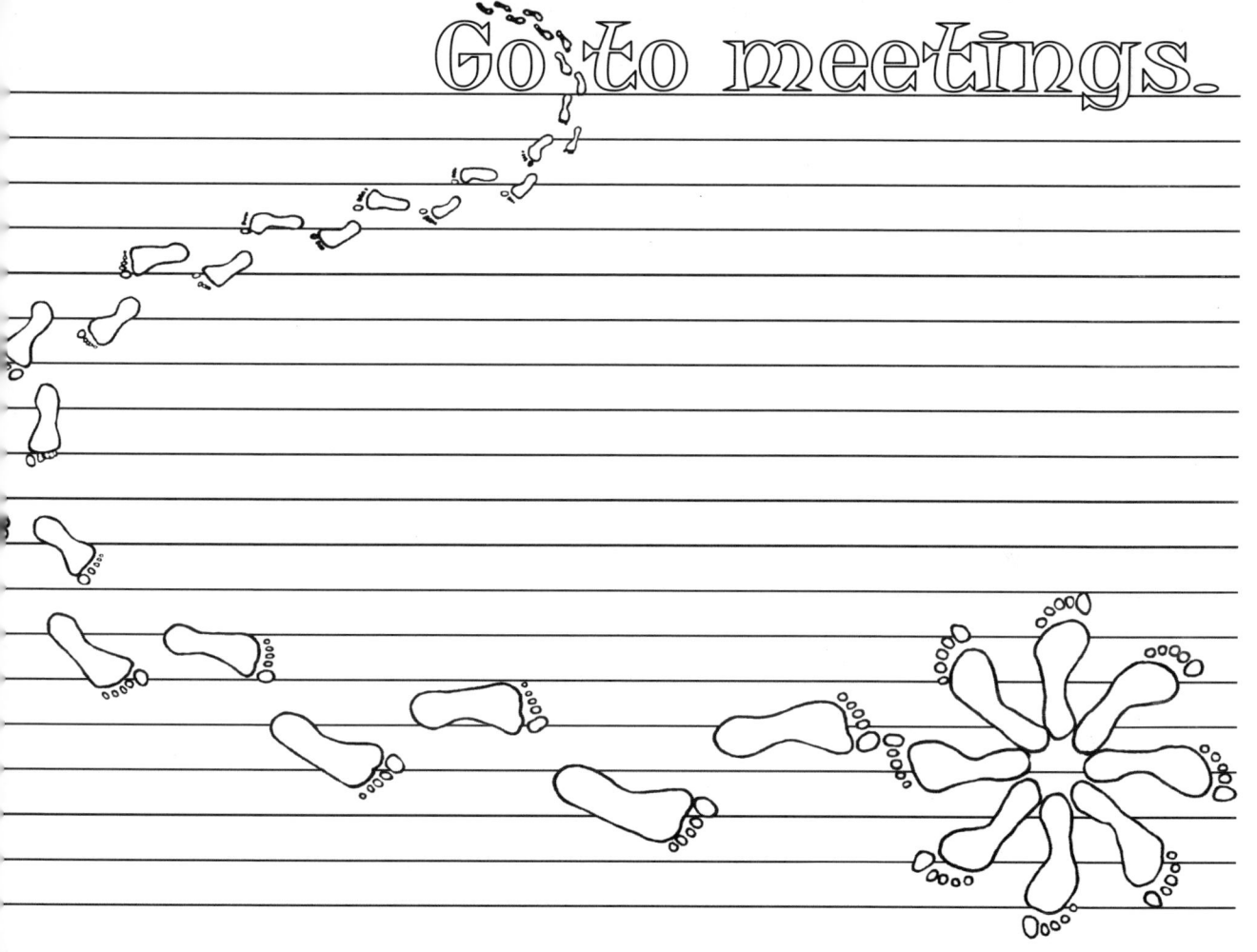

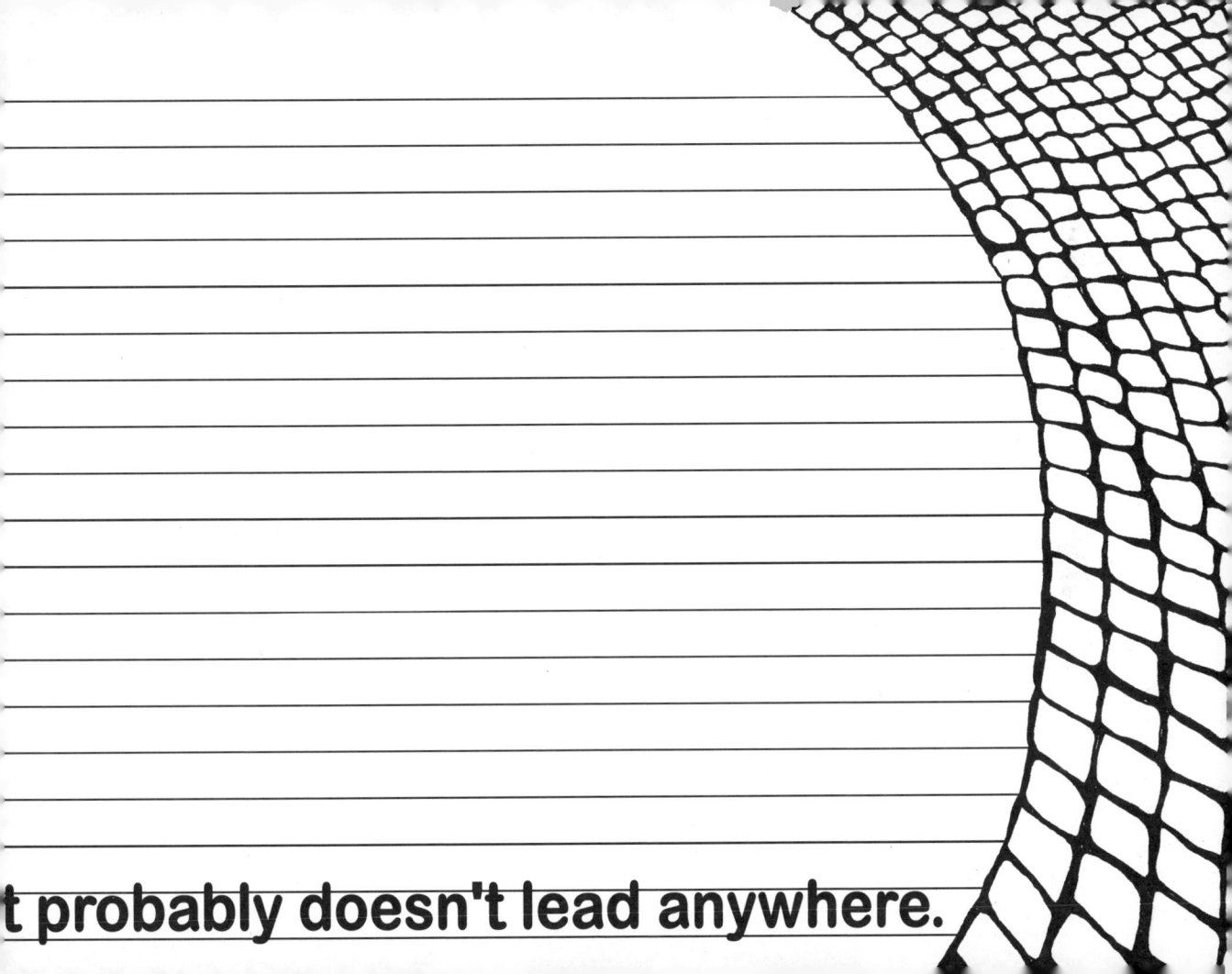

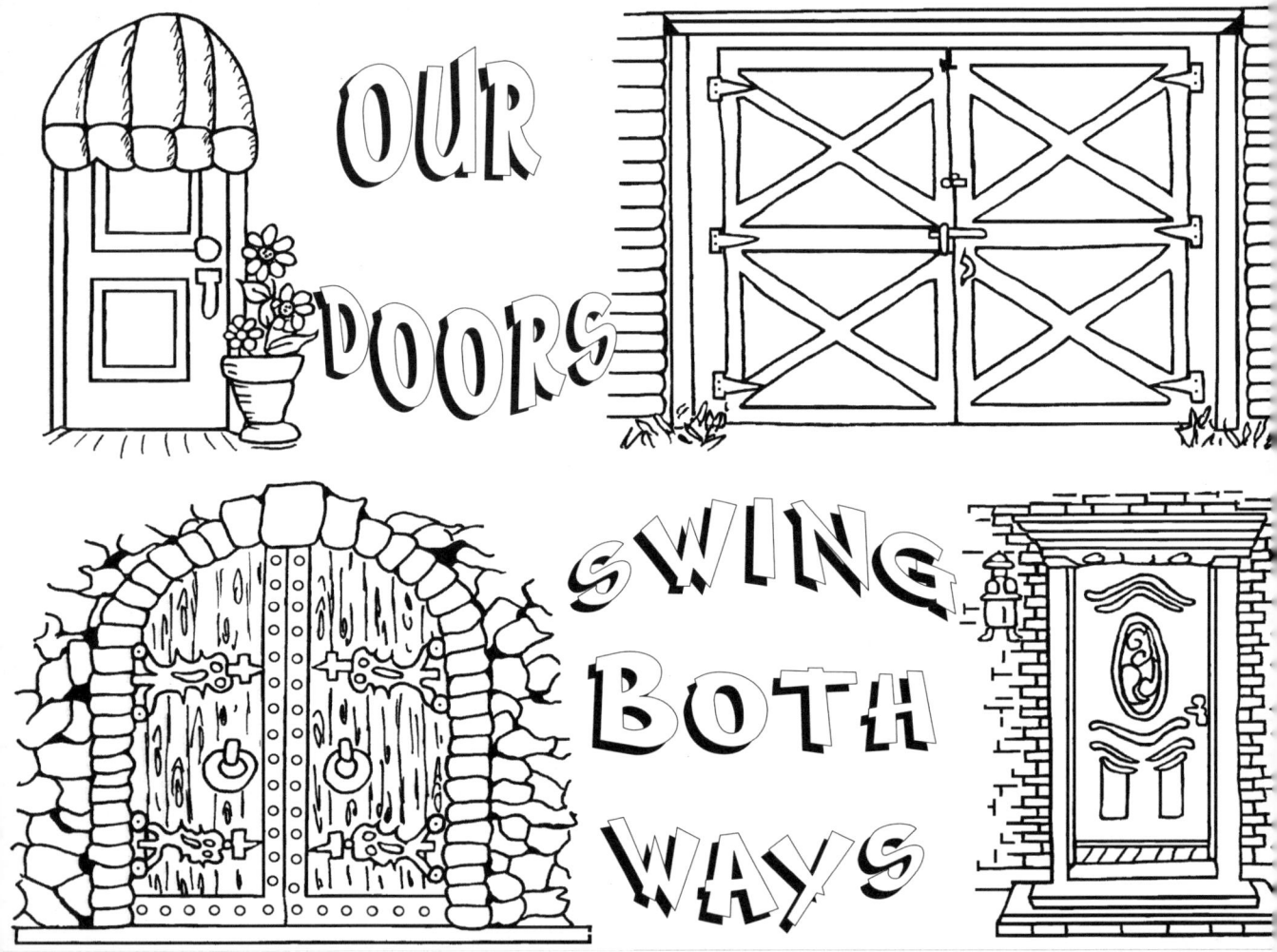

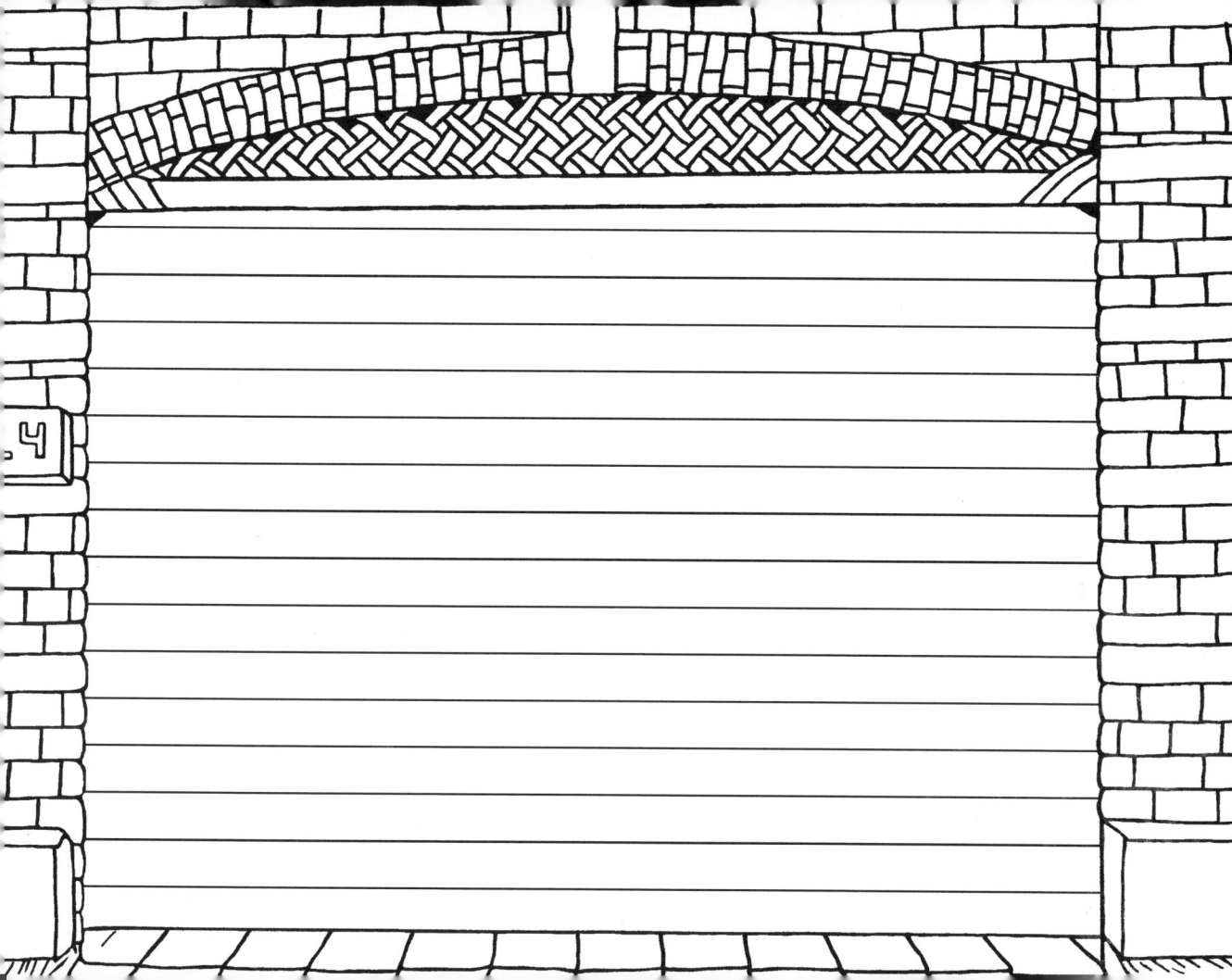

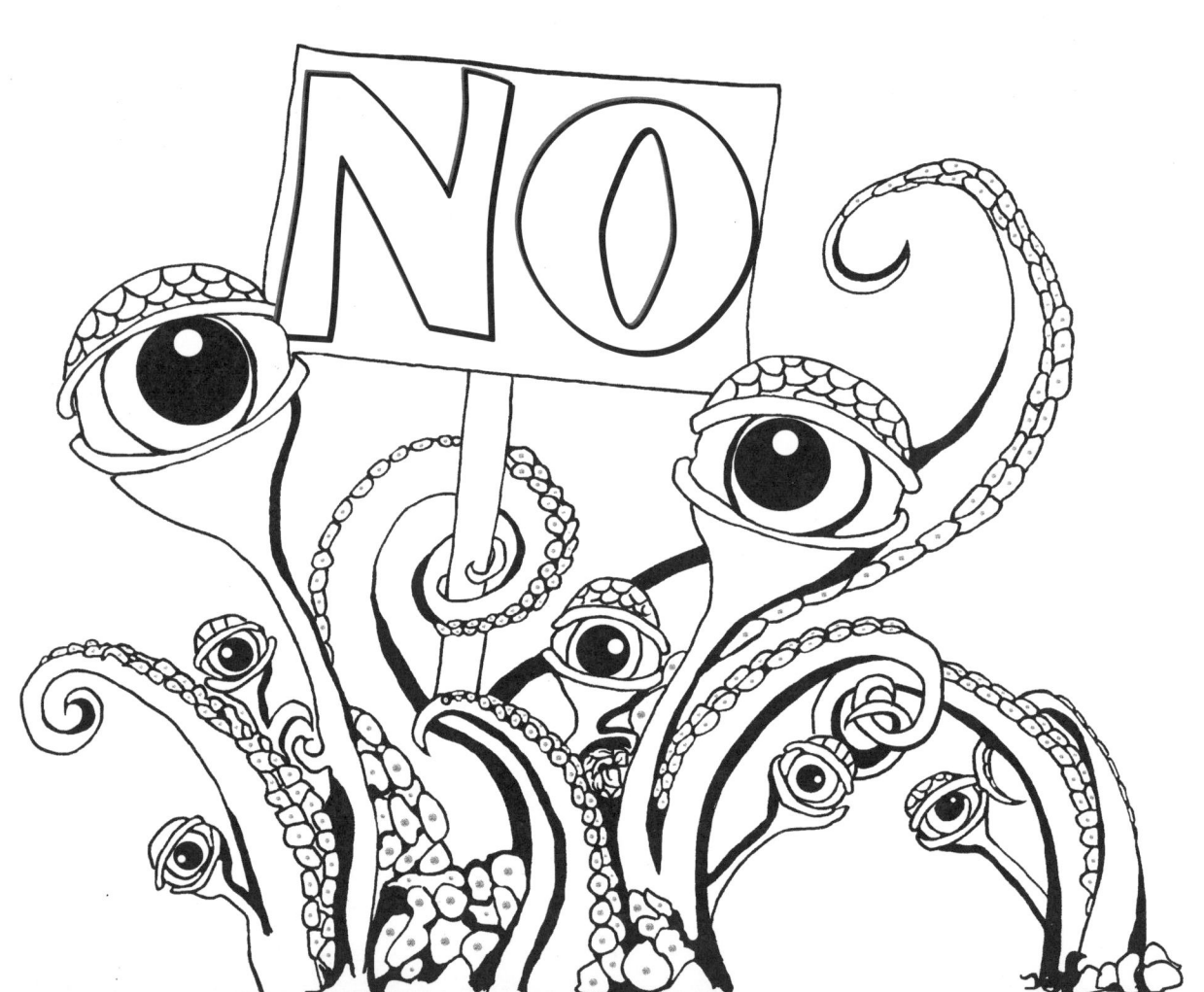

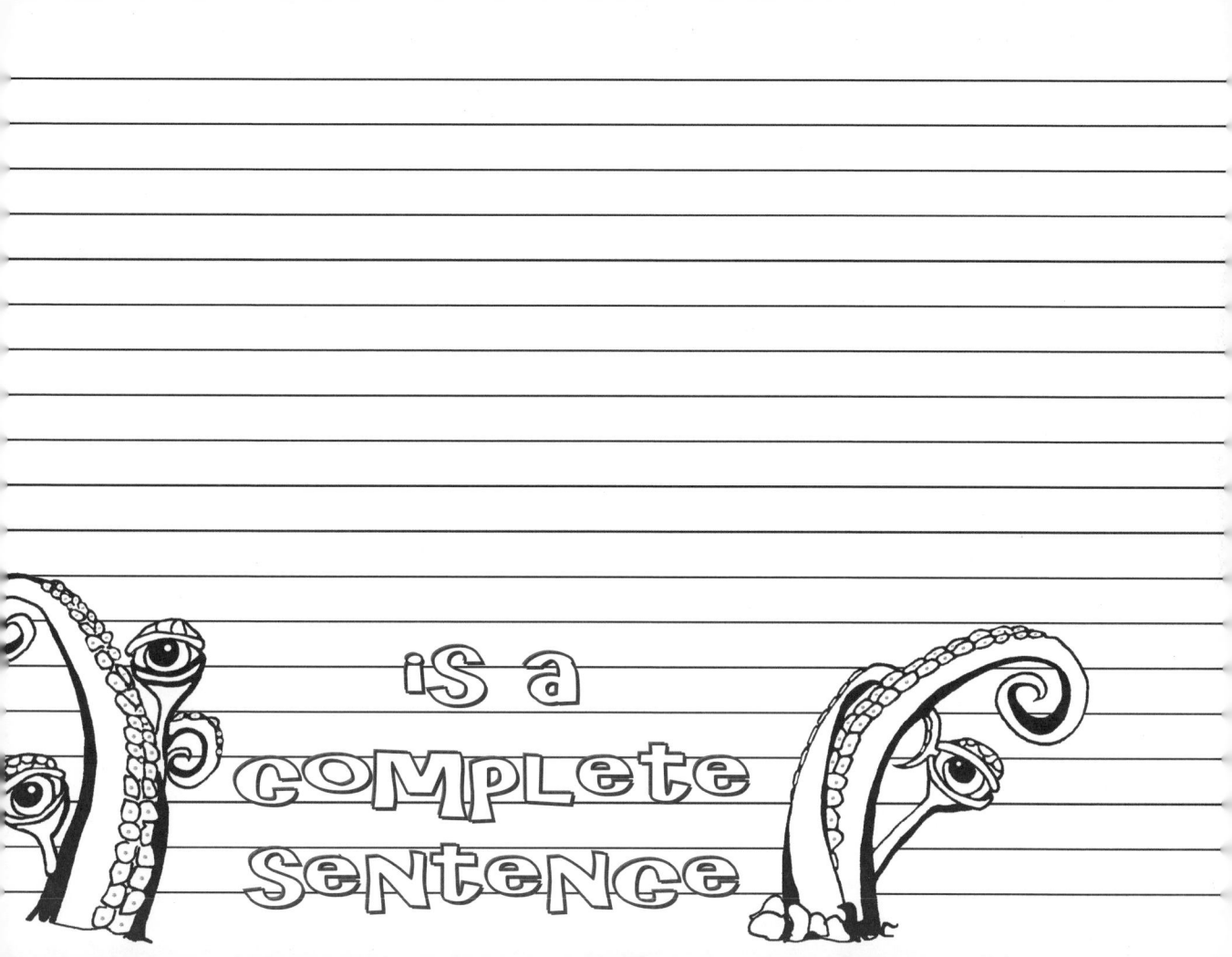

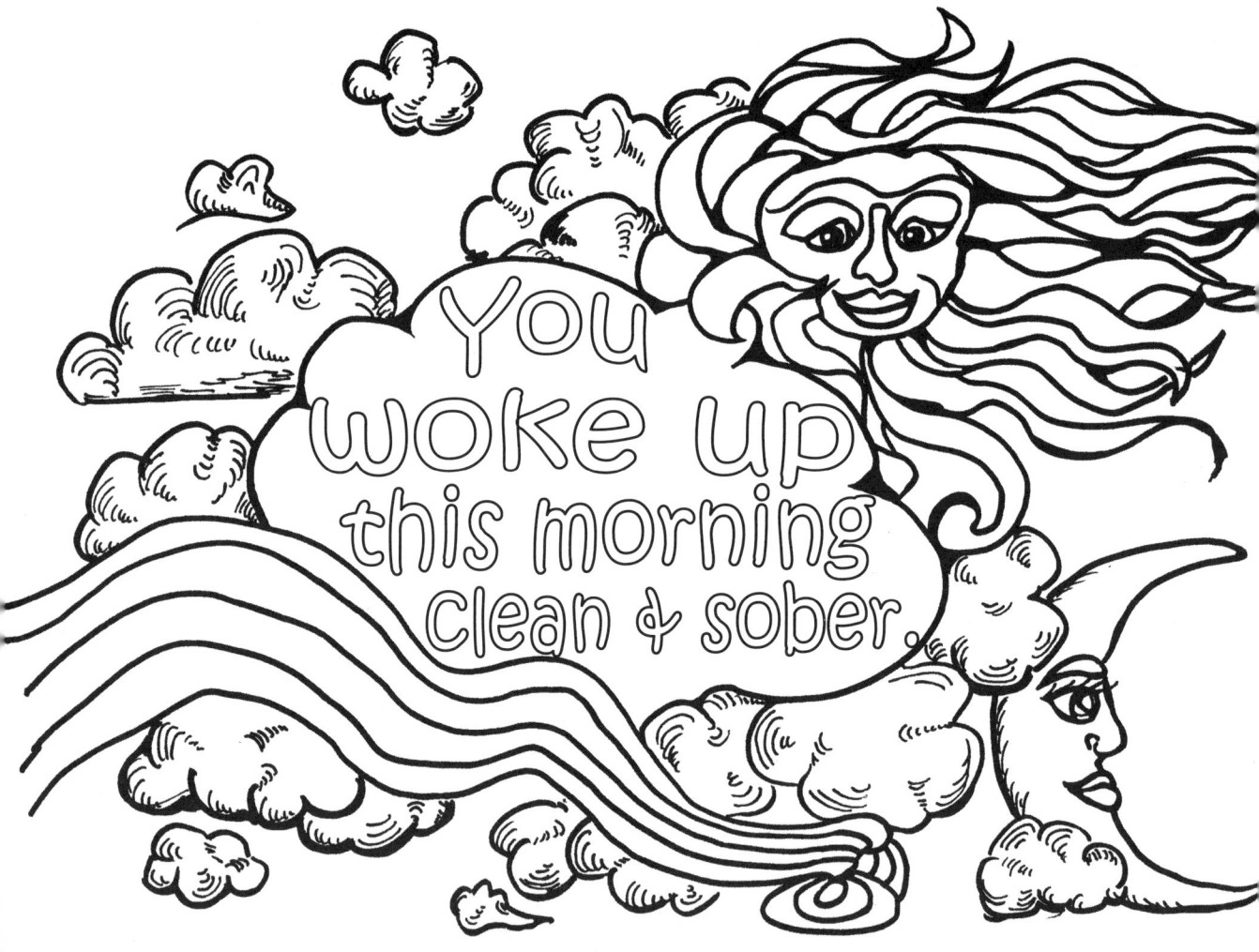

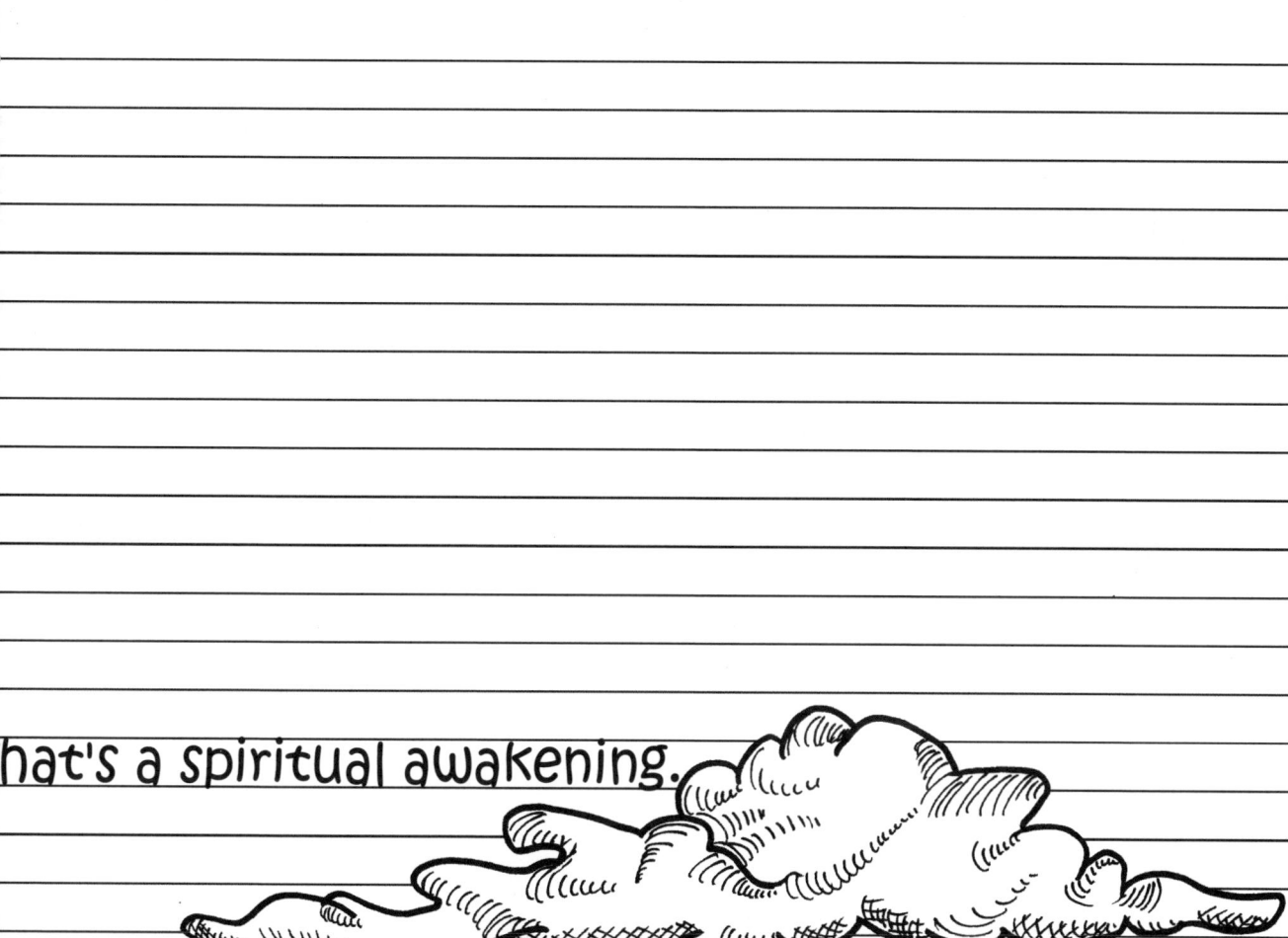

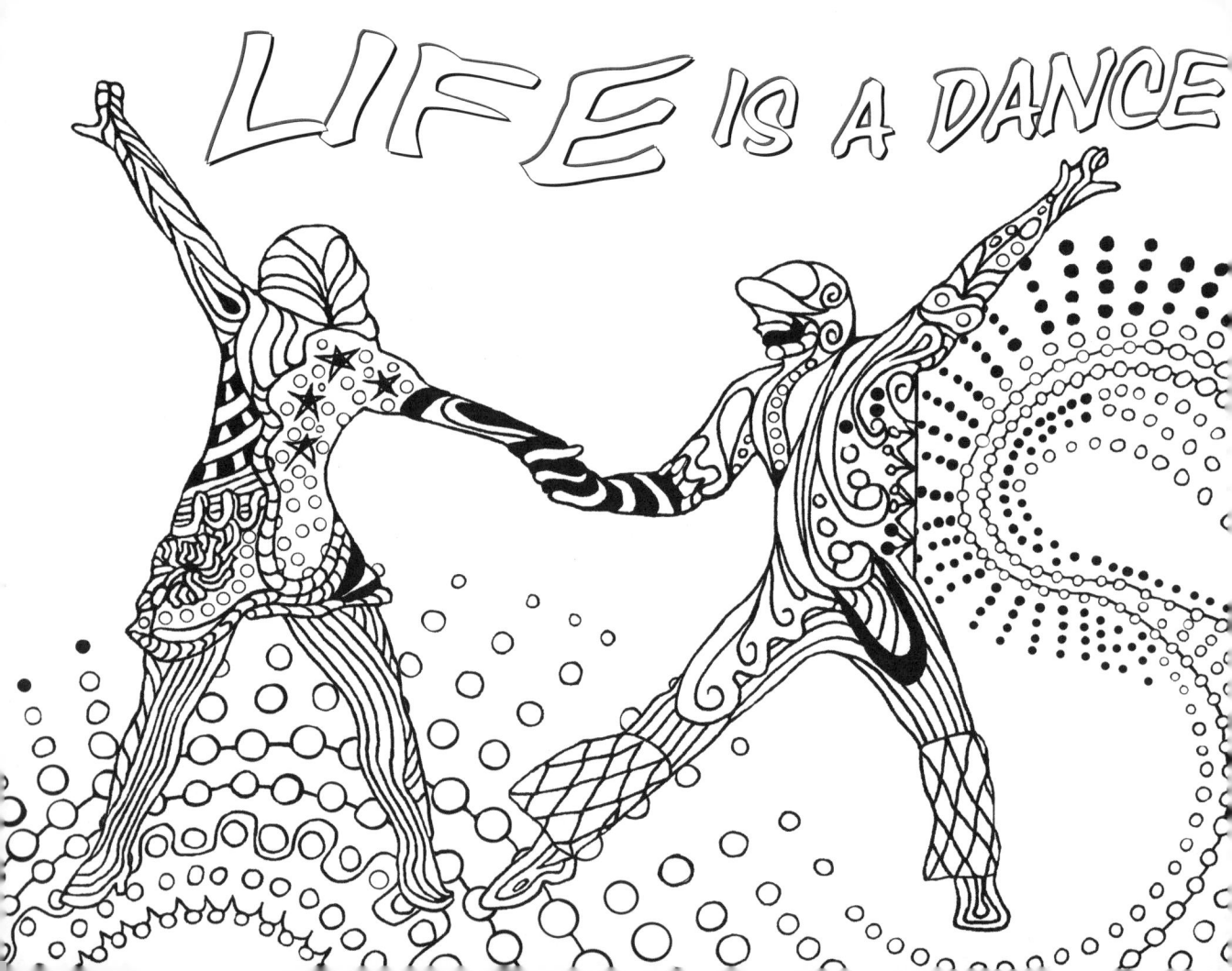

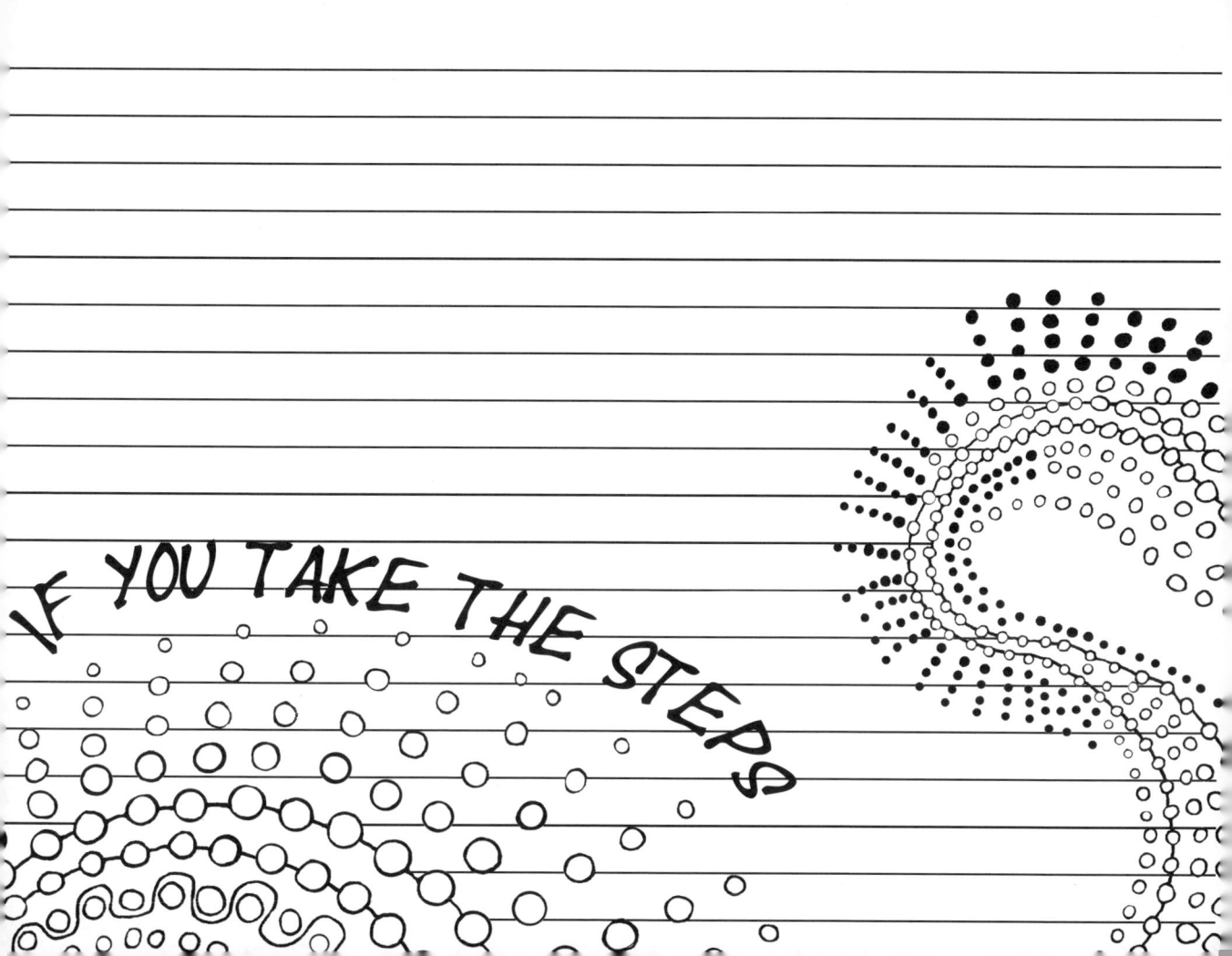

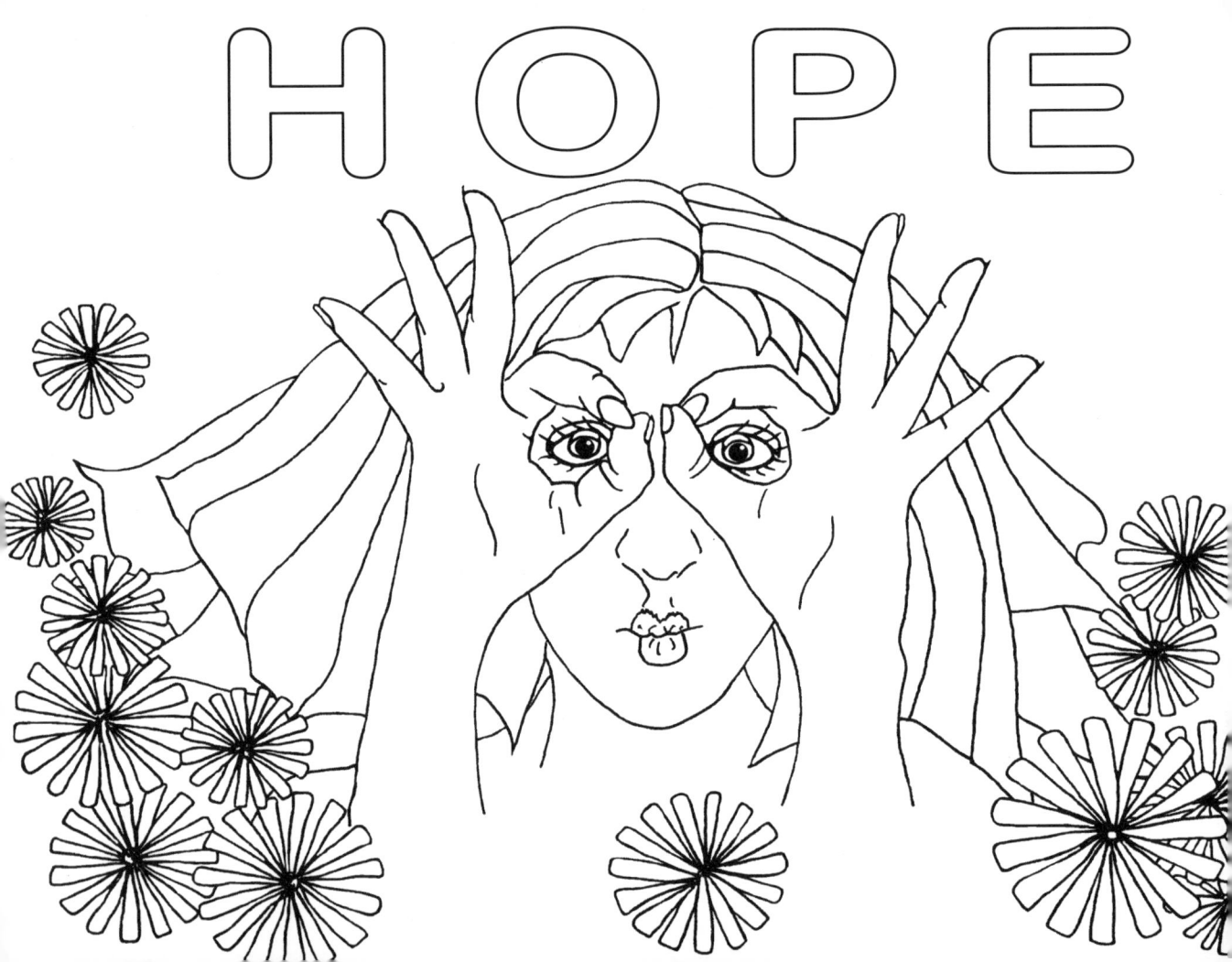

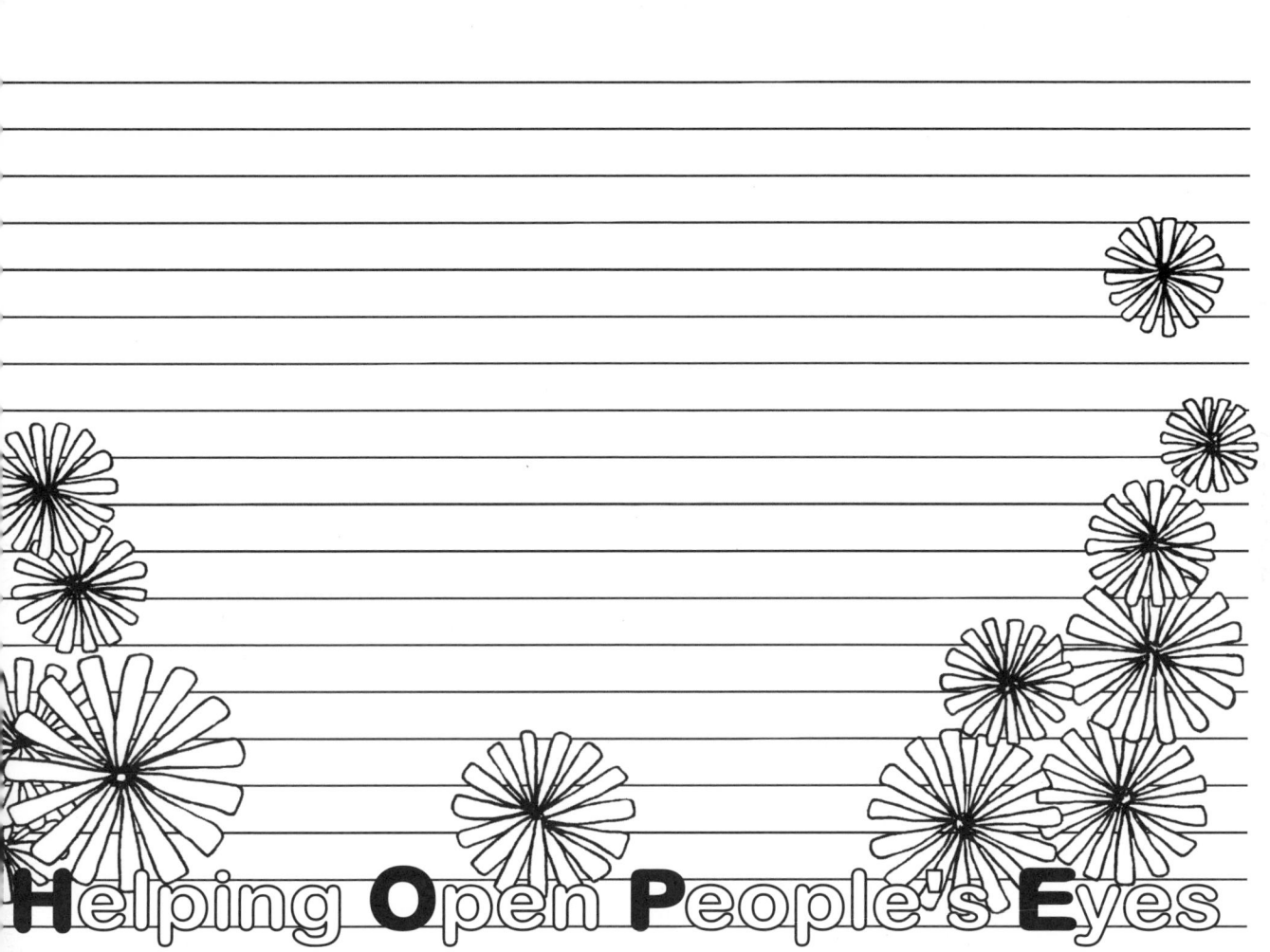

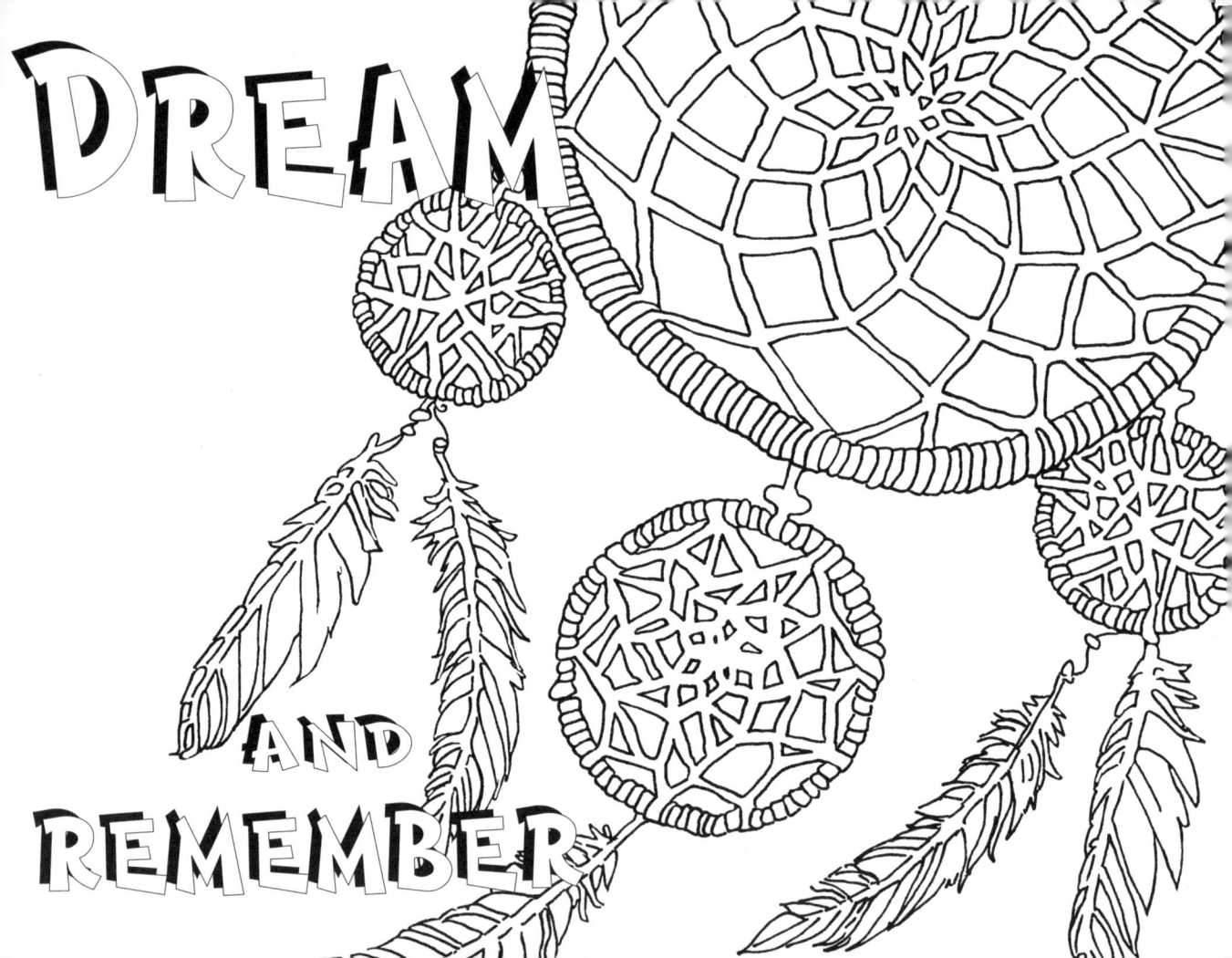

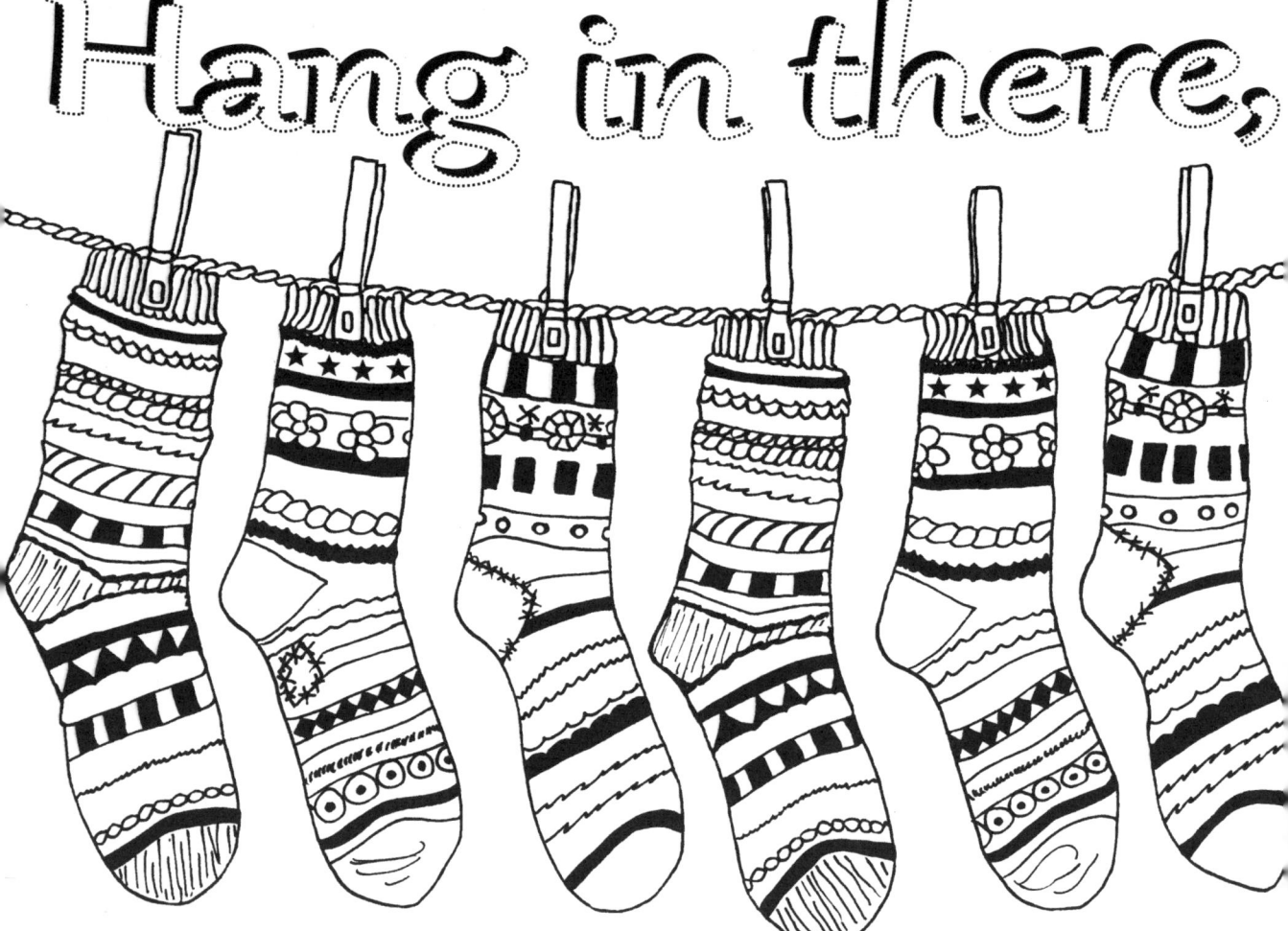

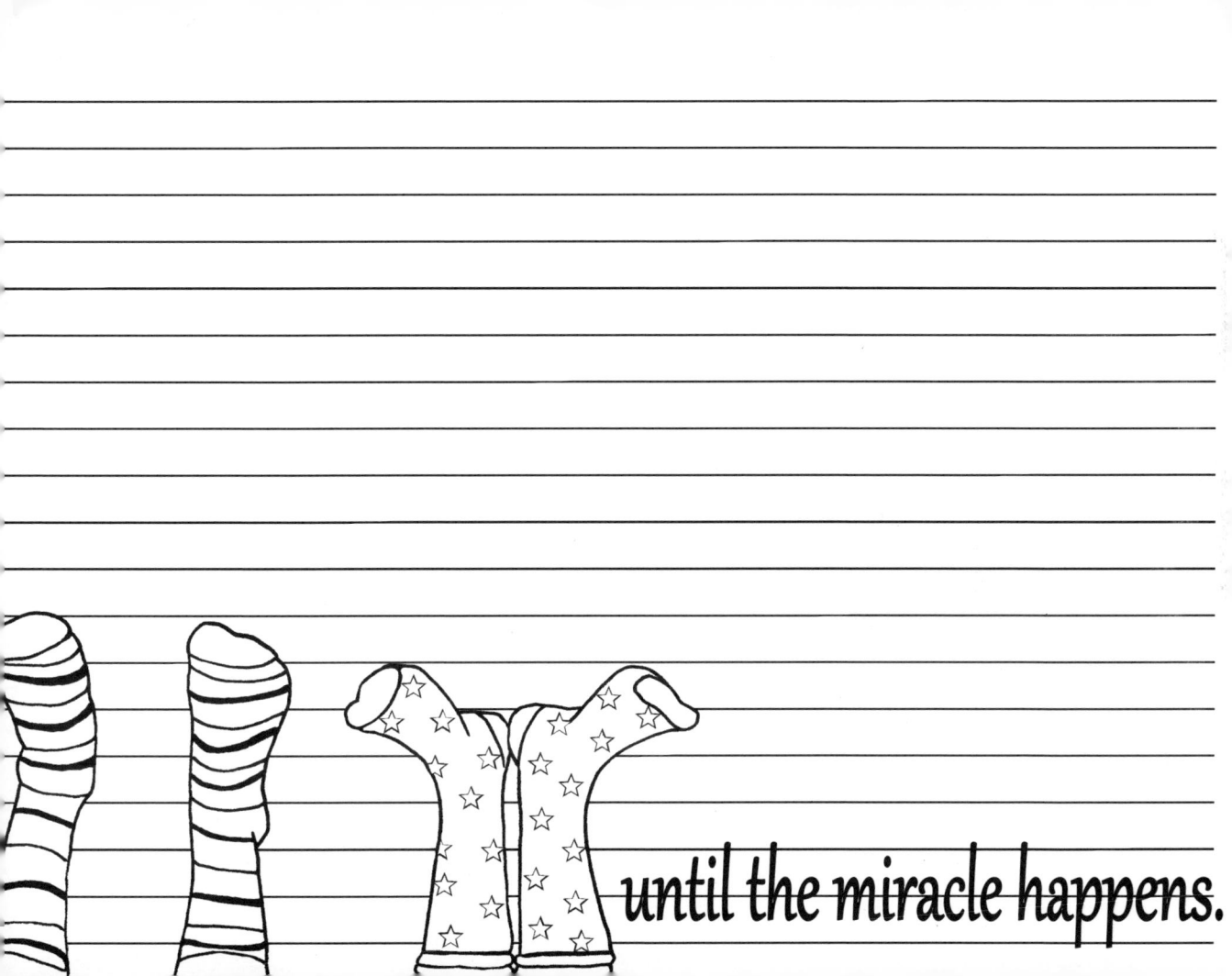
until the miracle happens.

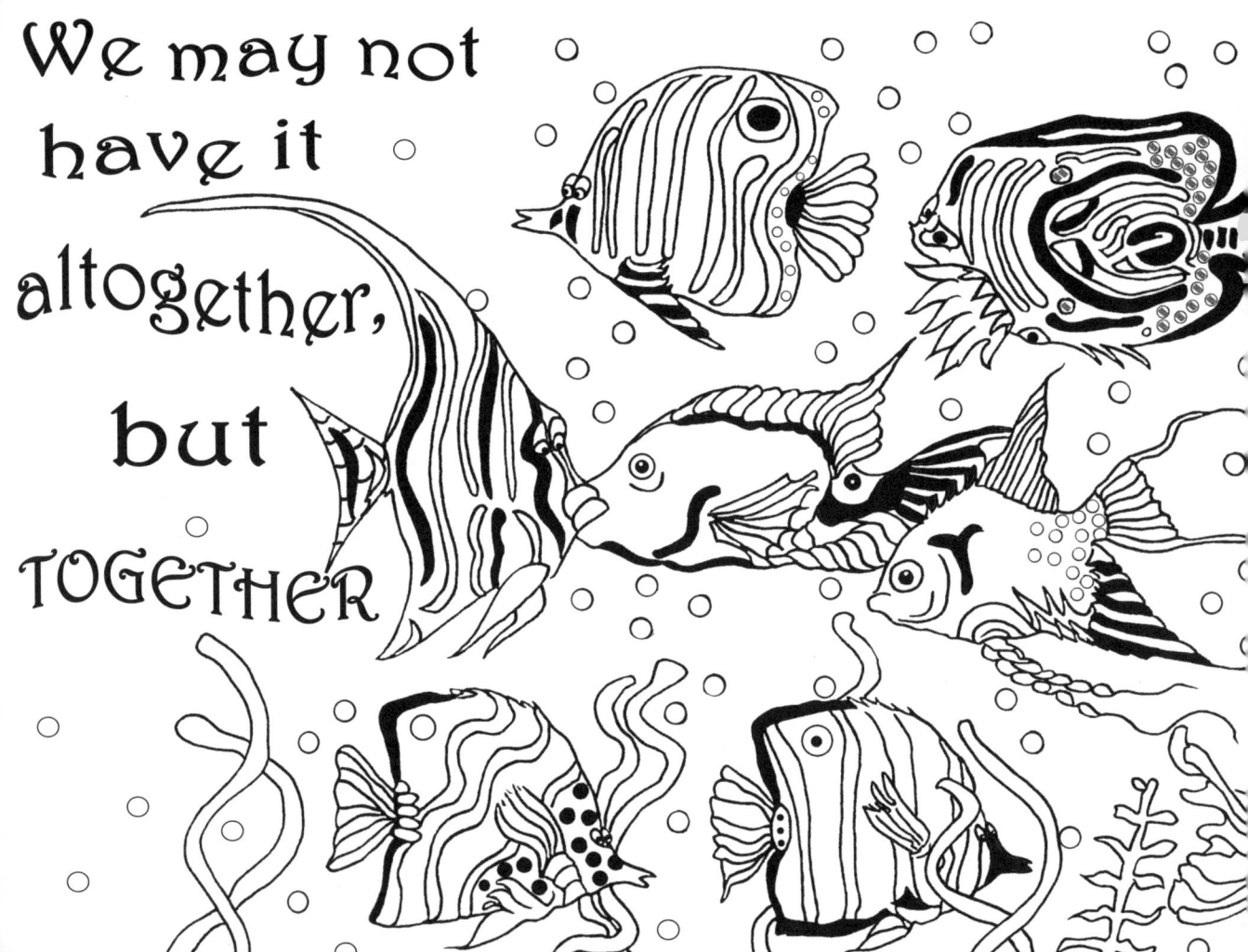

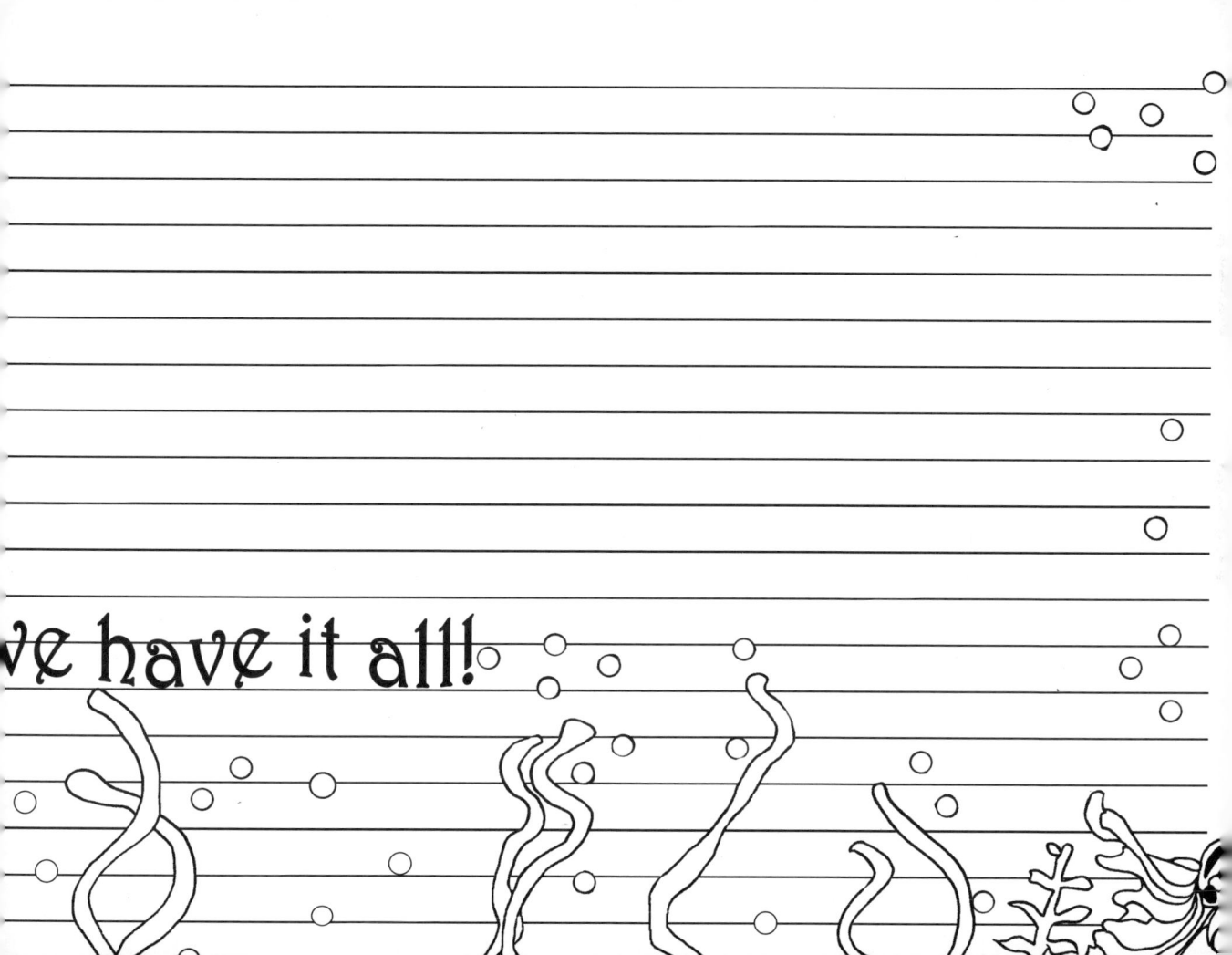

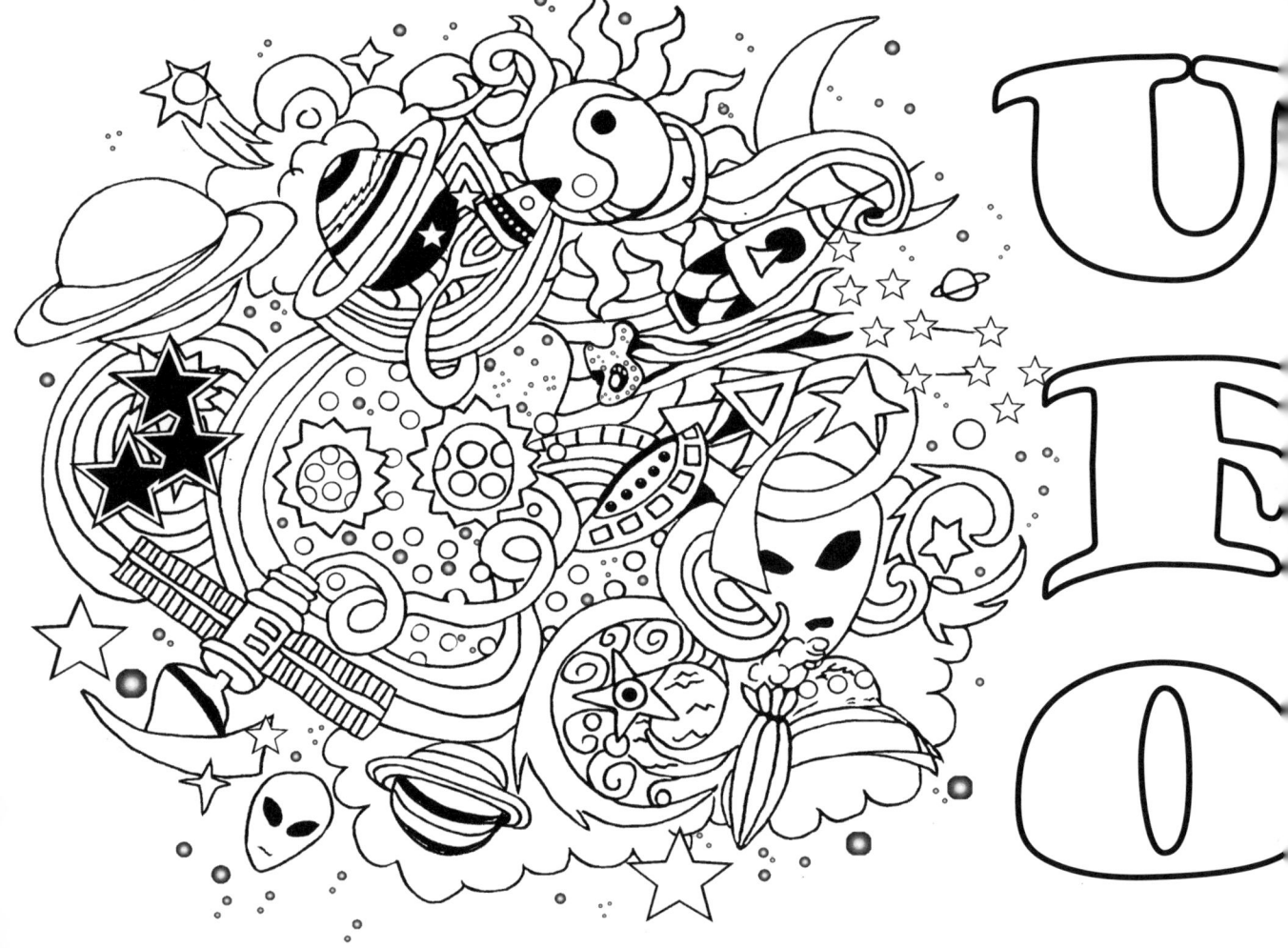

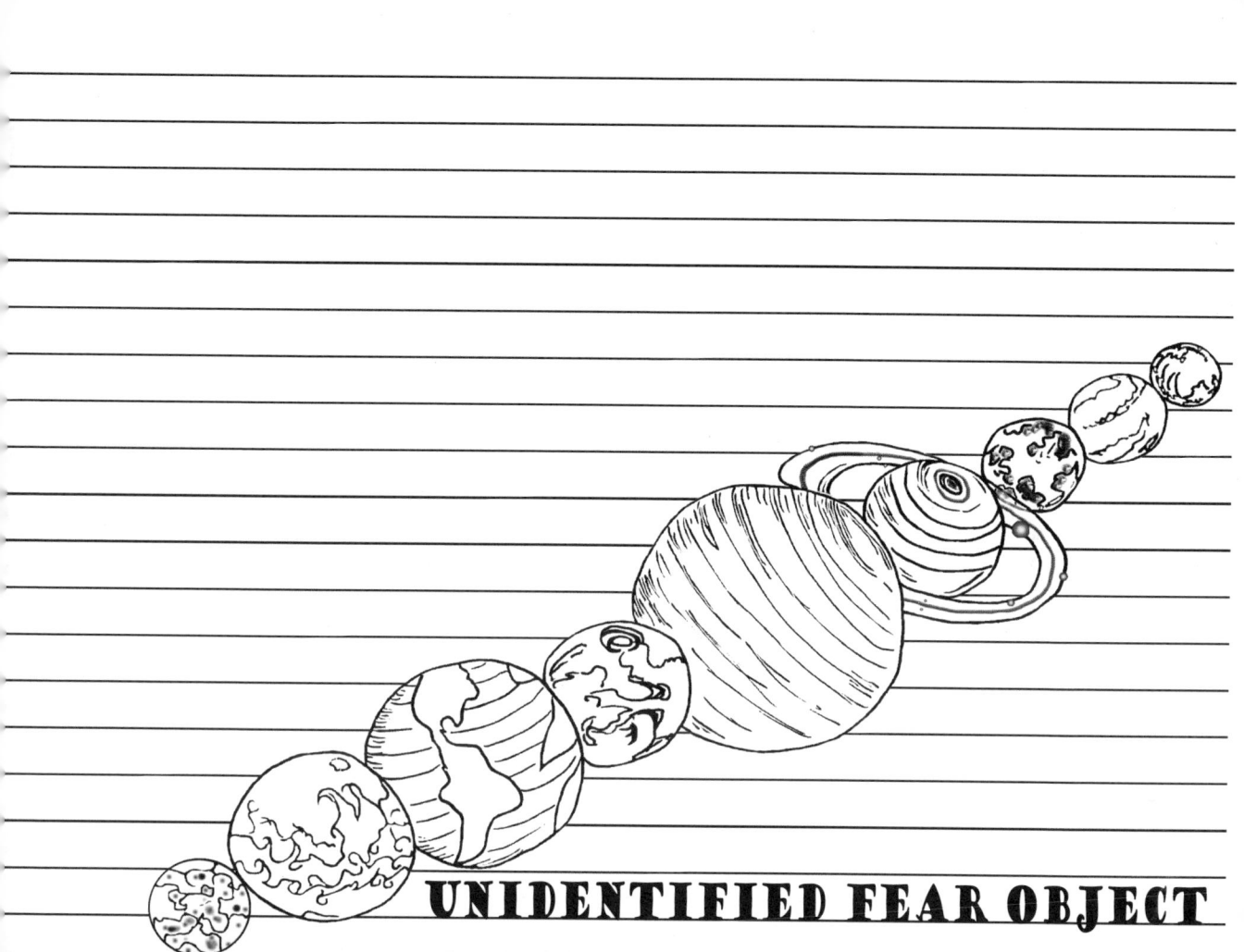

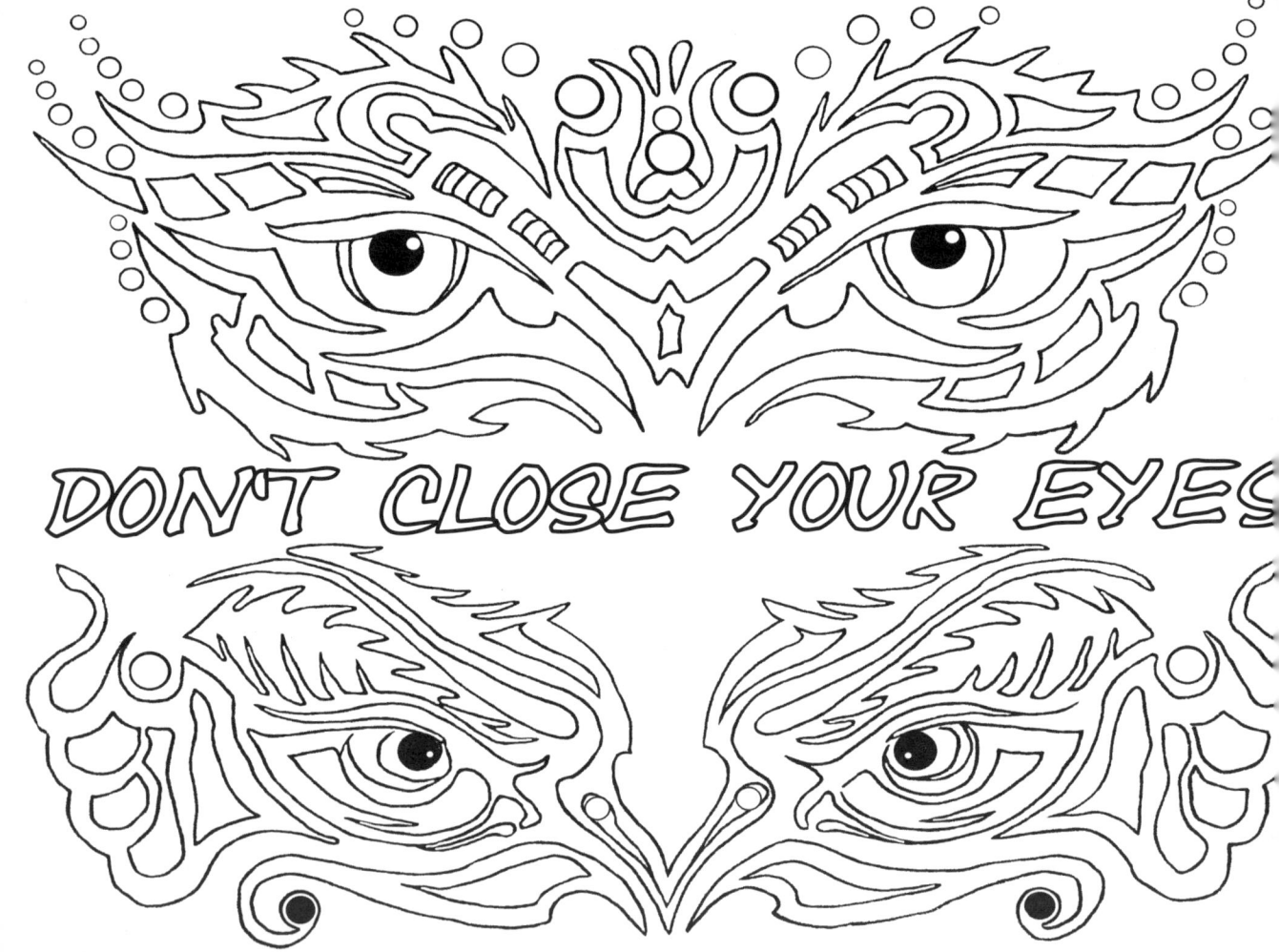

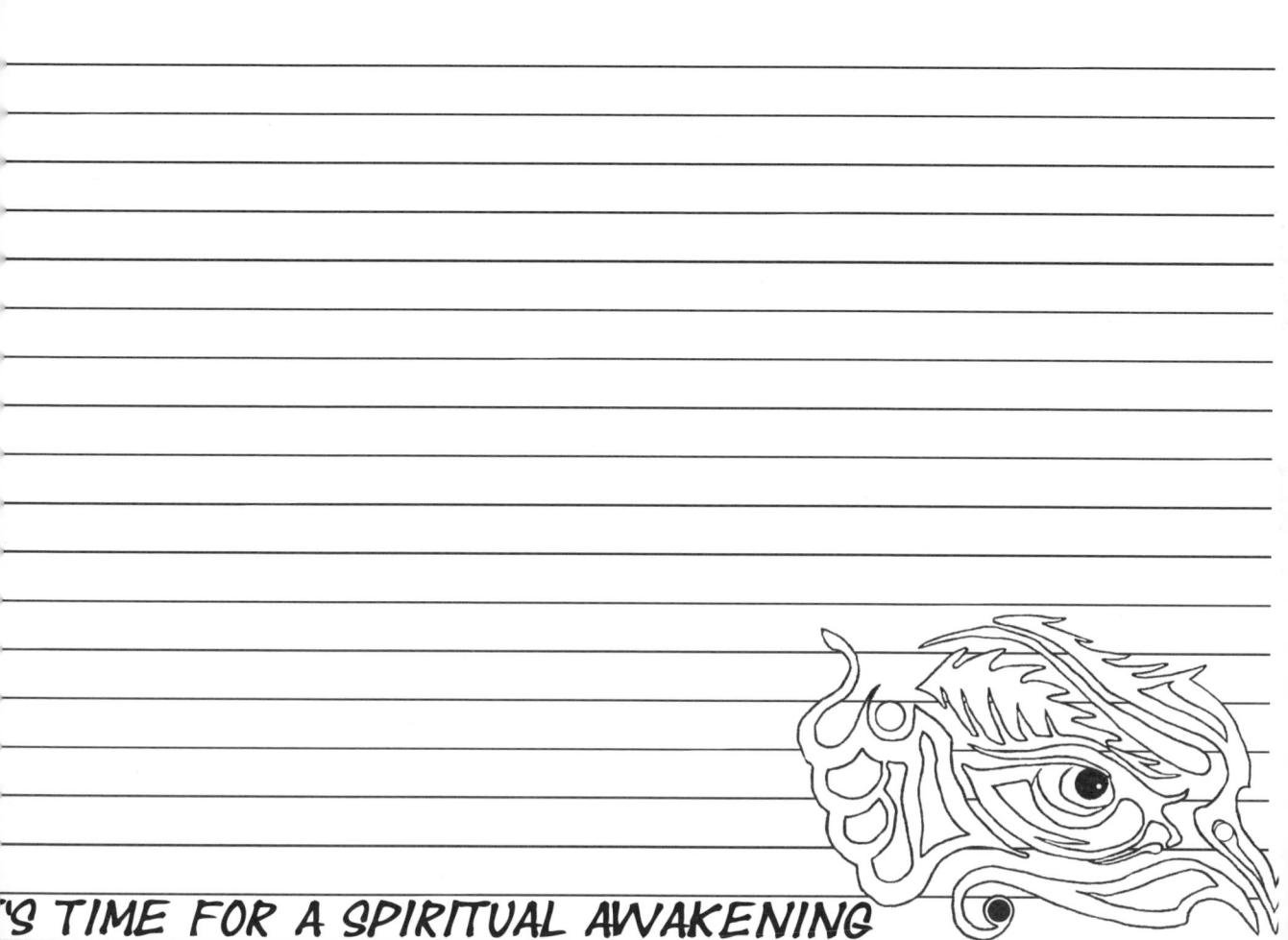

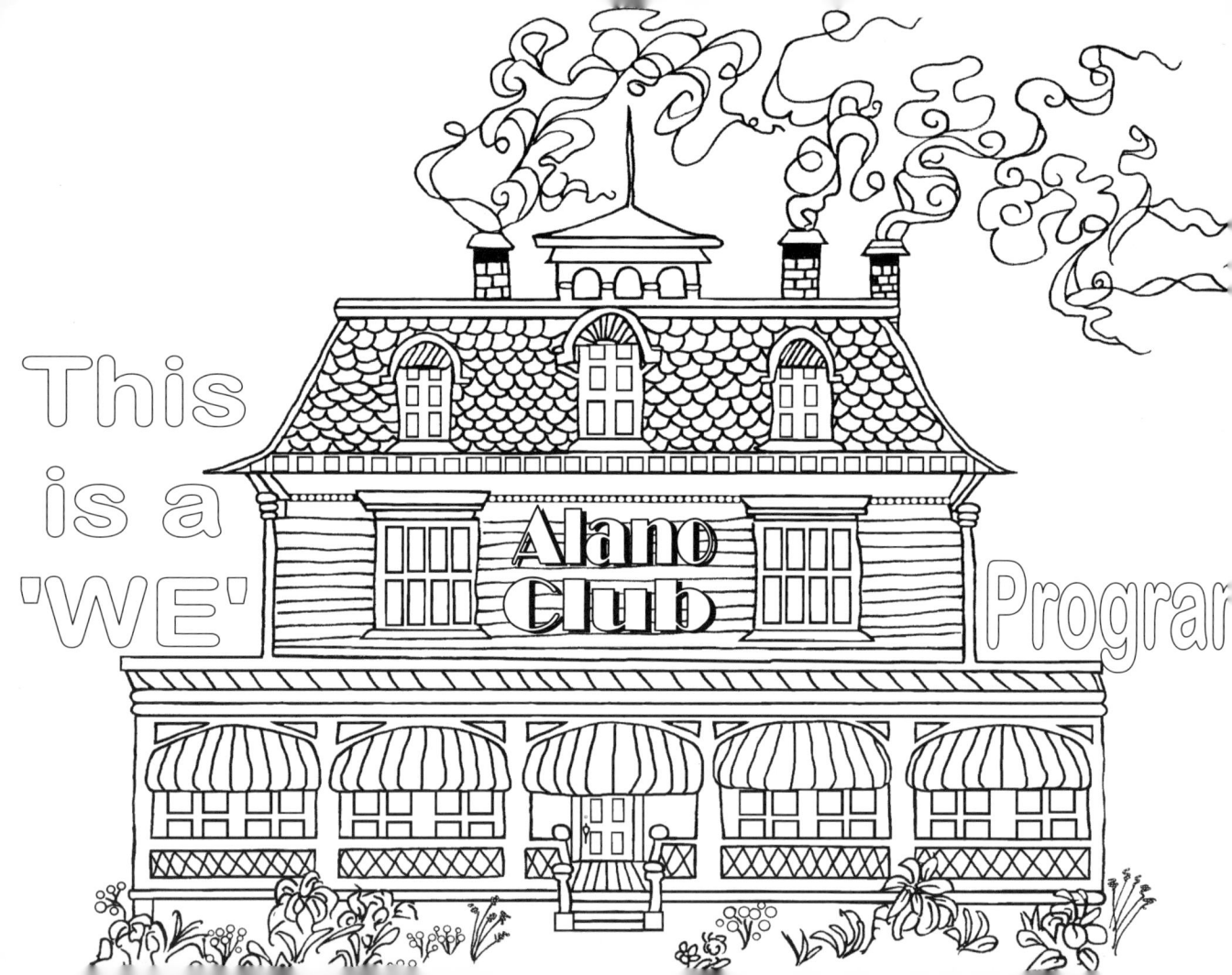

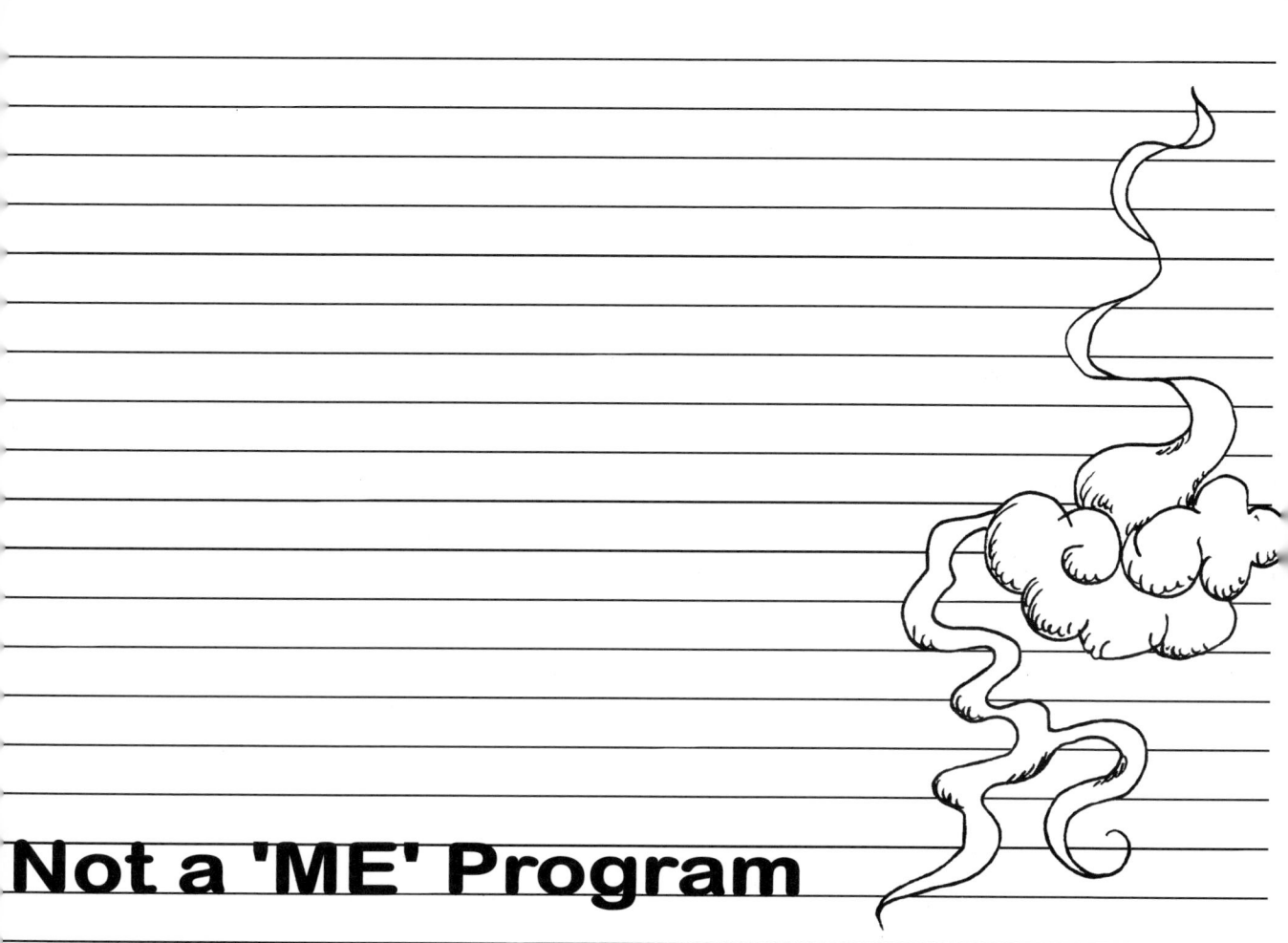

Not a 'ME' Program

Go to Meetings to Listen

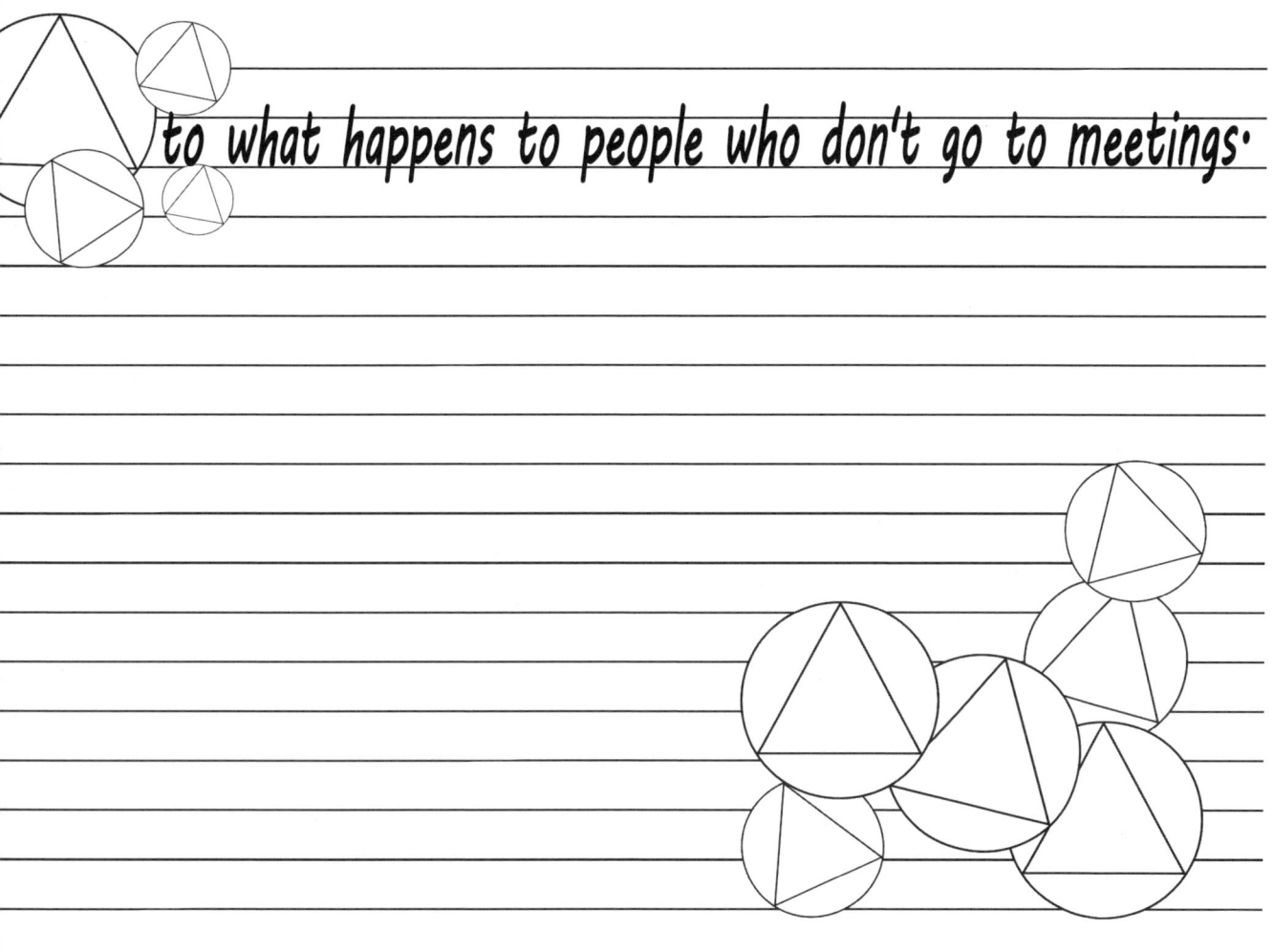
to what happens to people who don't go to meetings.

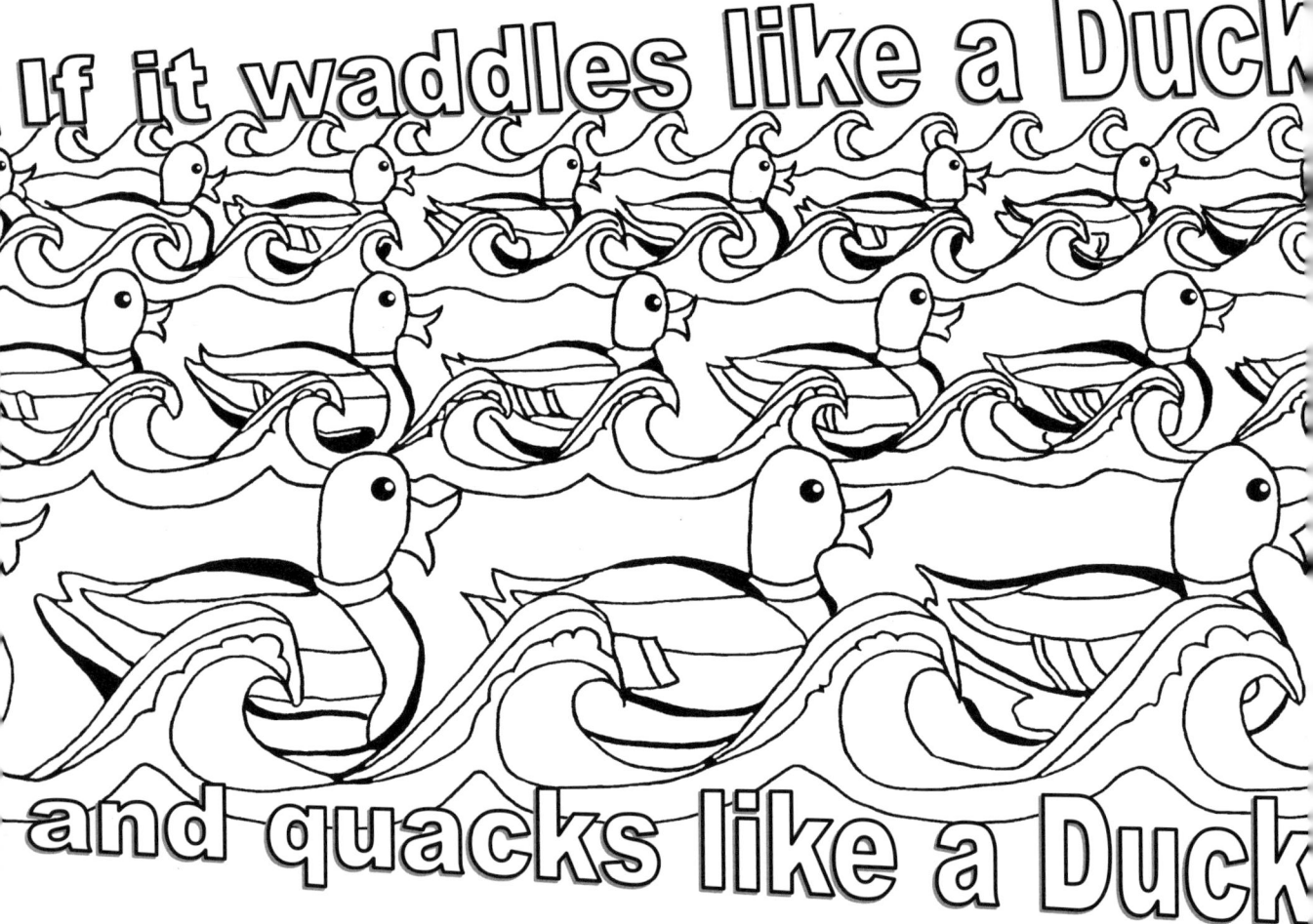

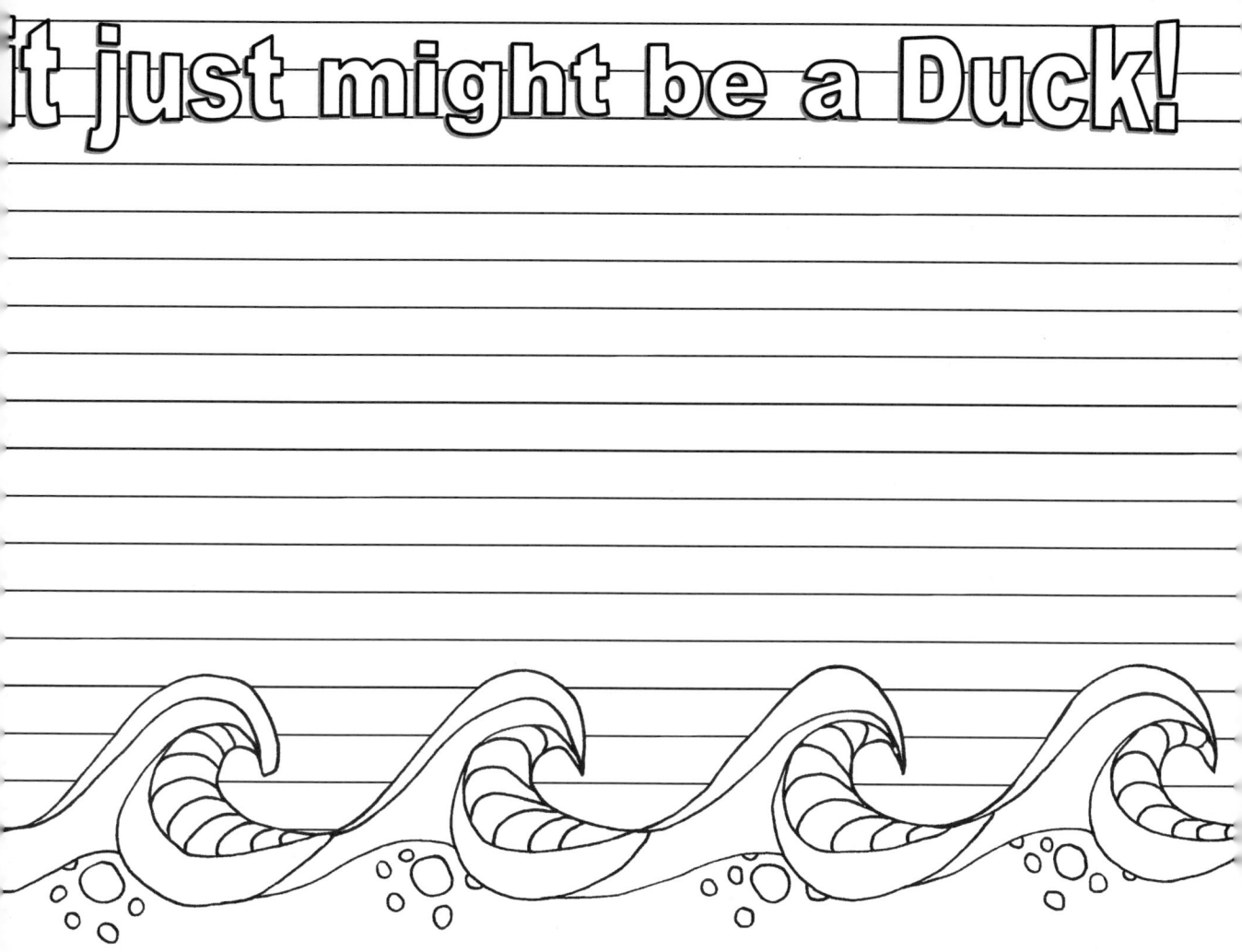

I work toward becoming the person

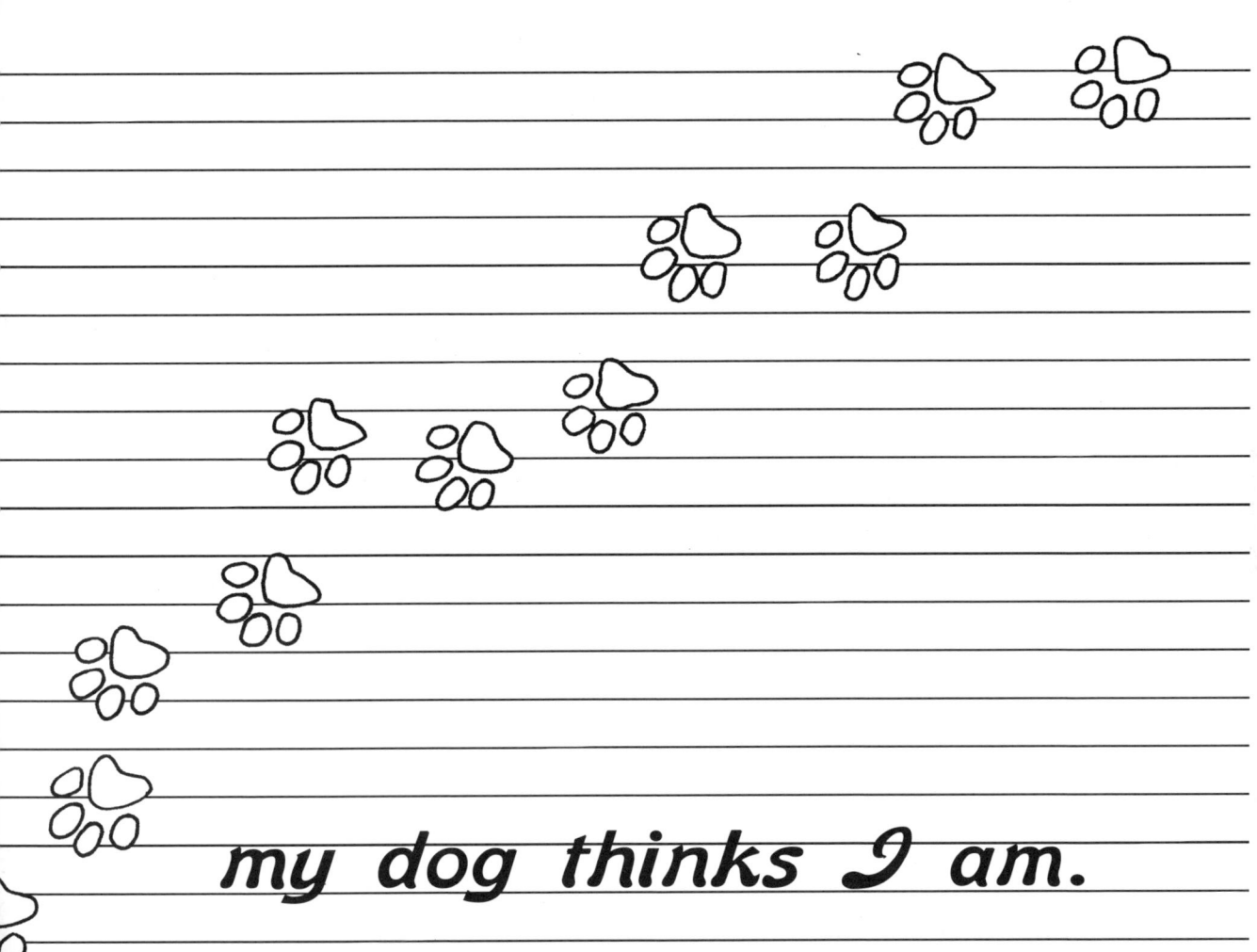

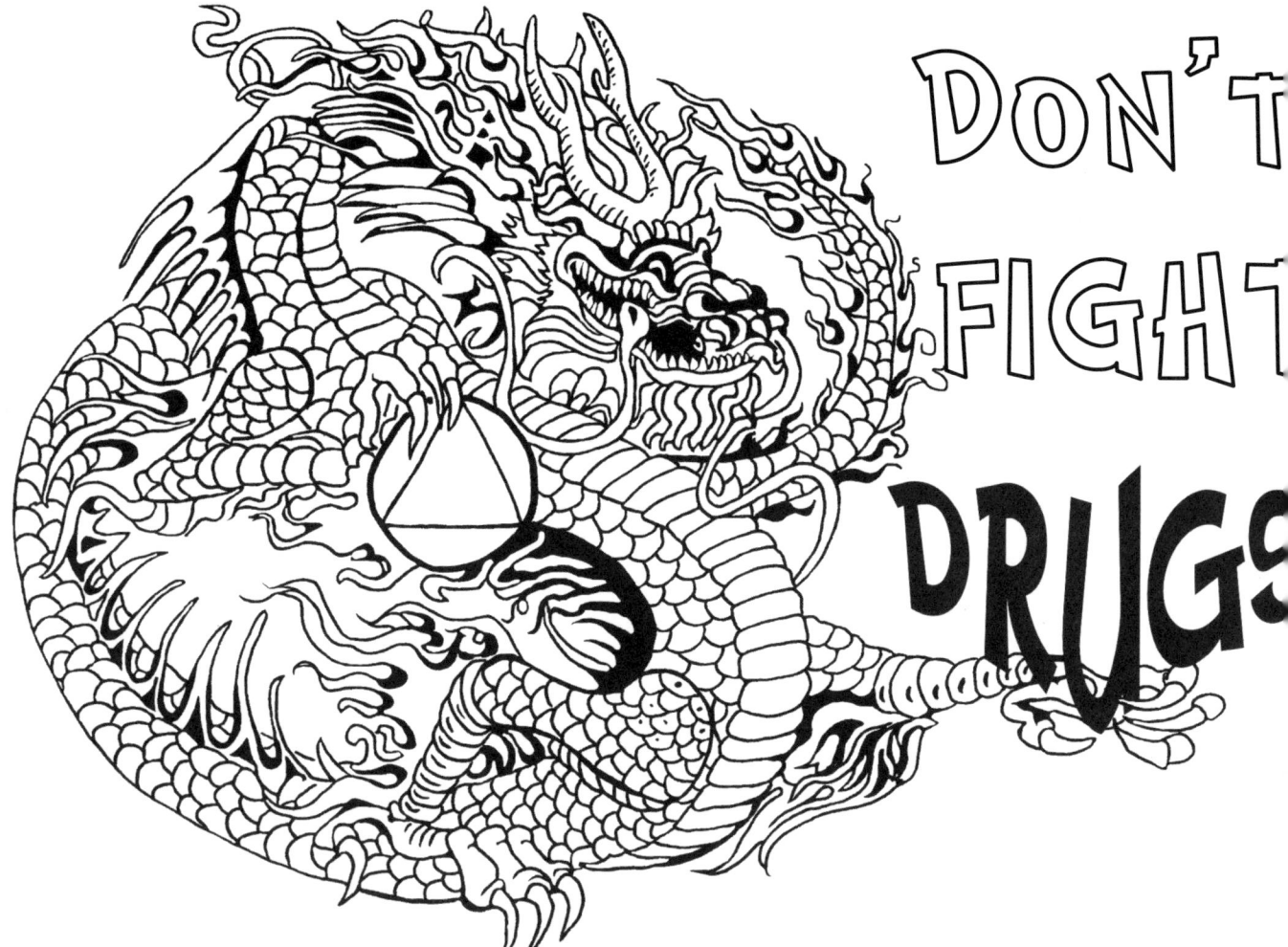

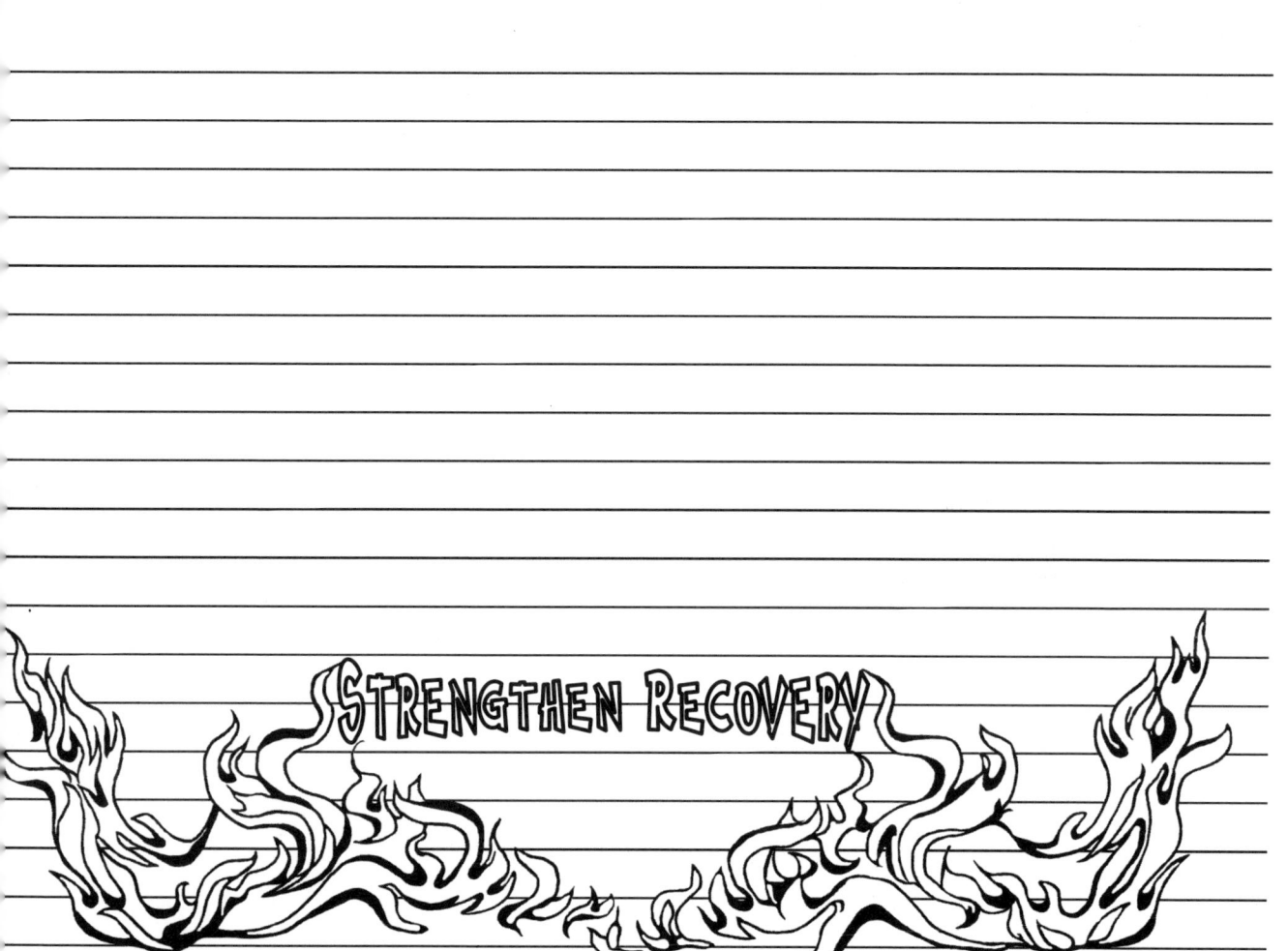

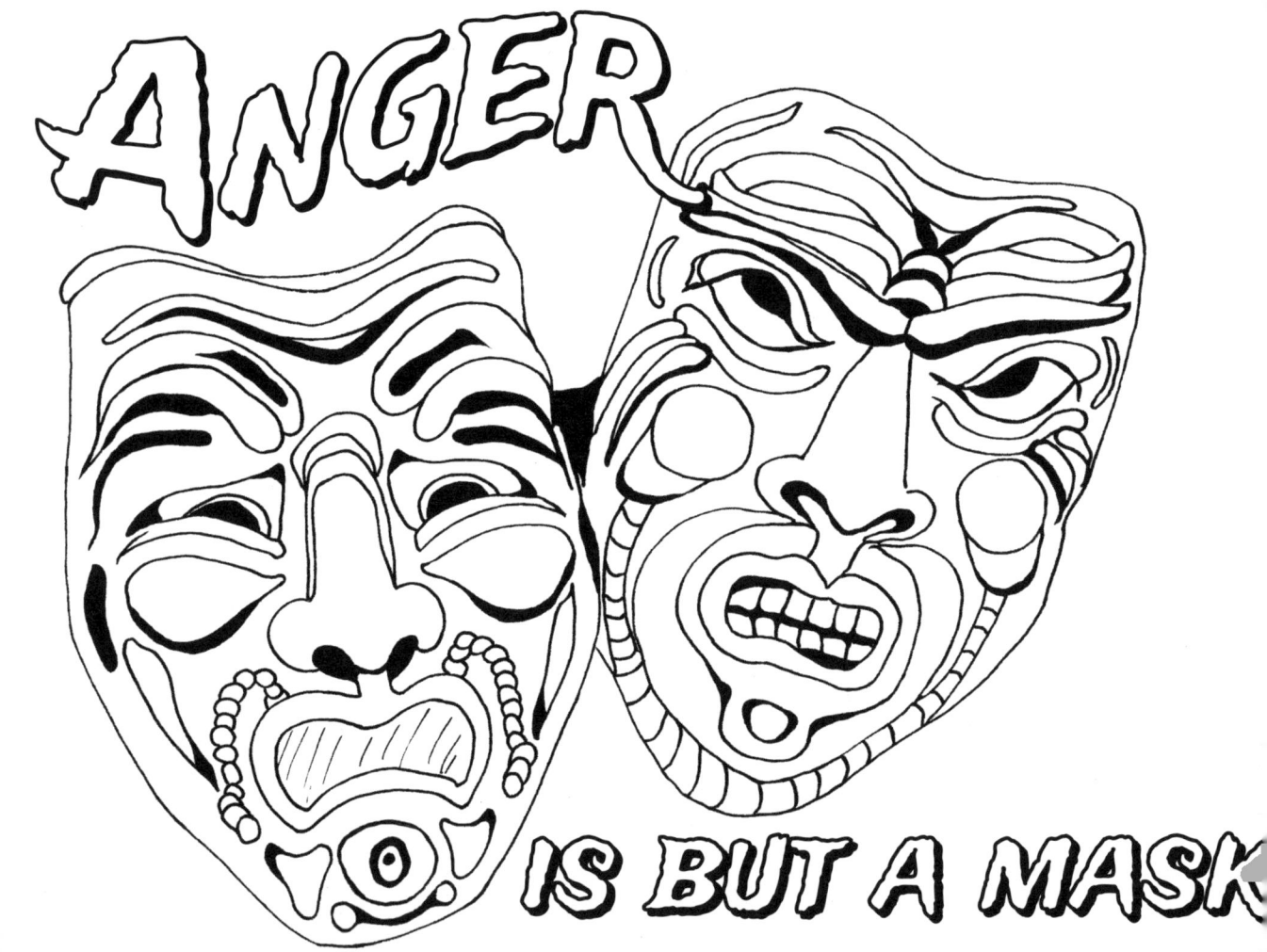

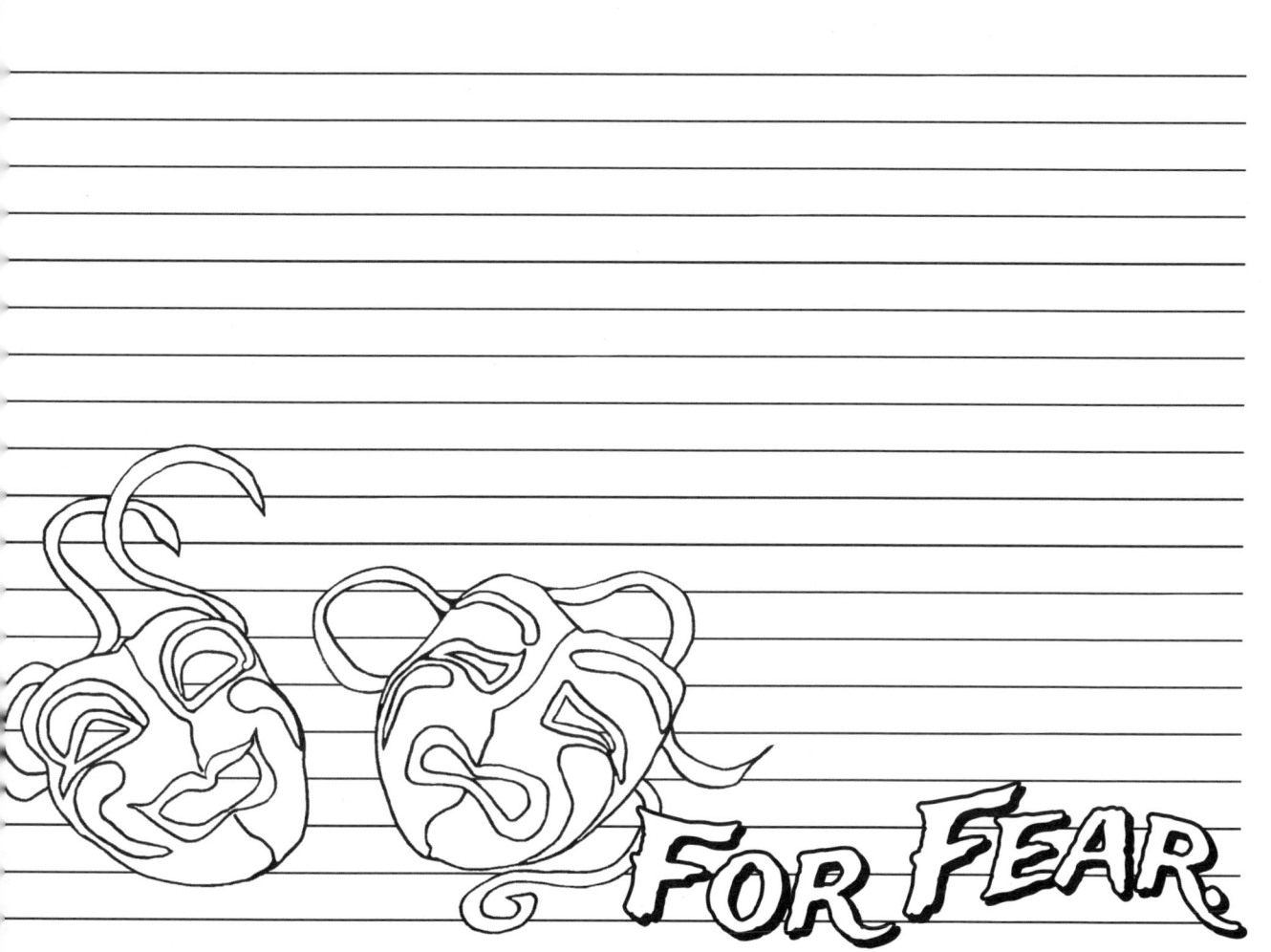

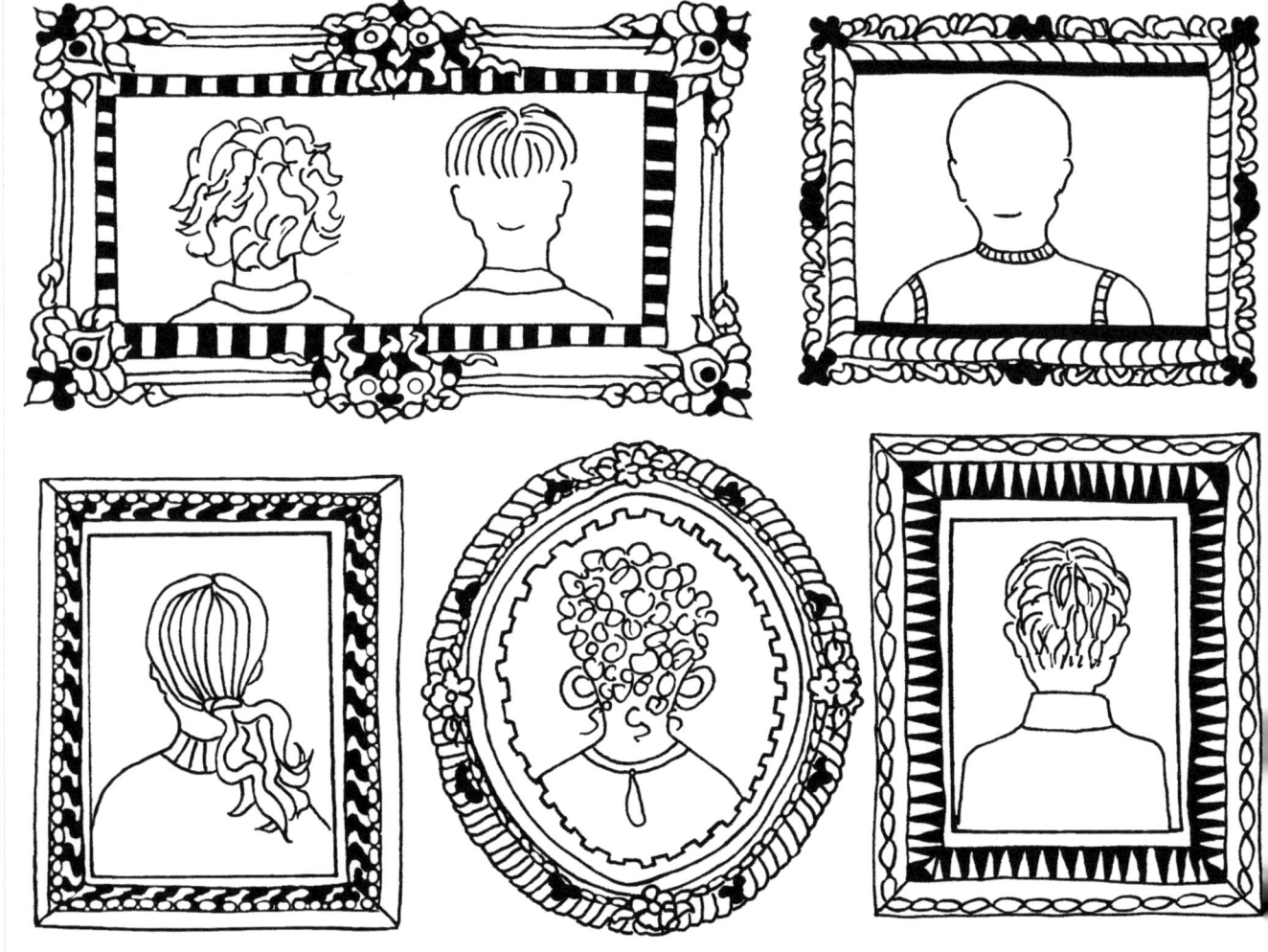

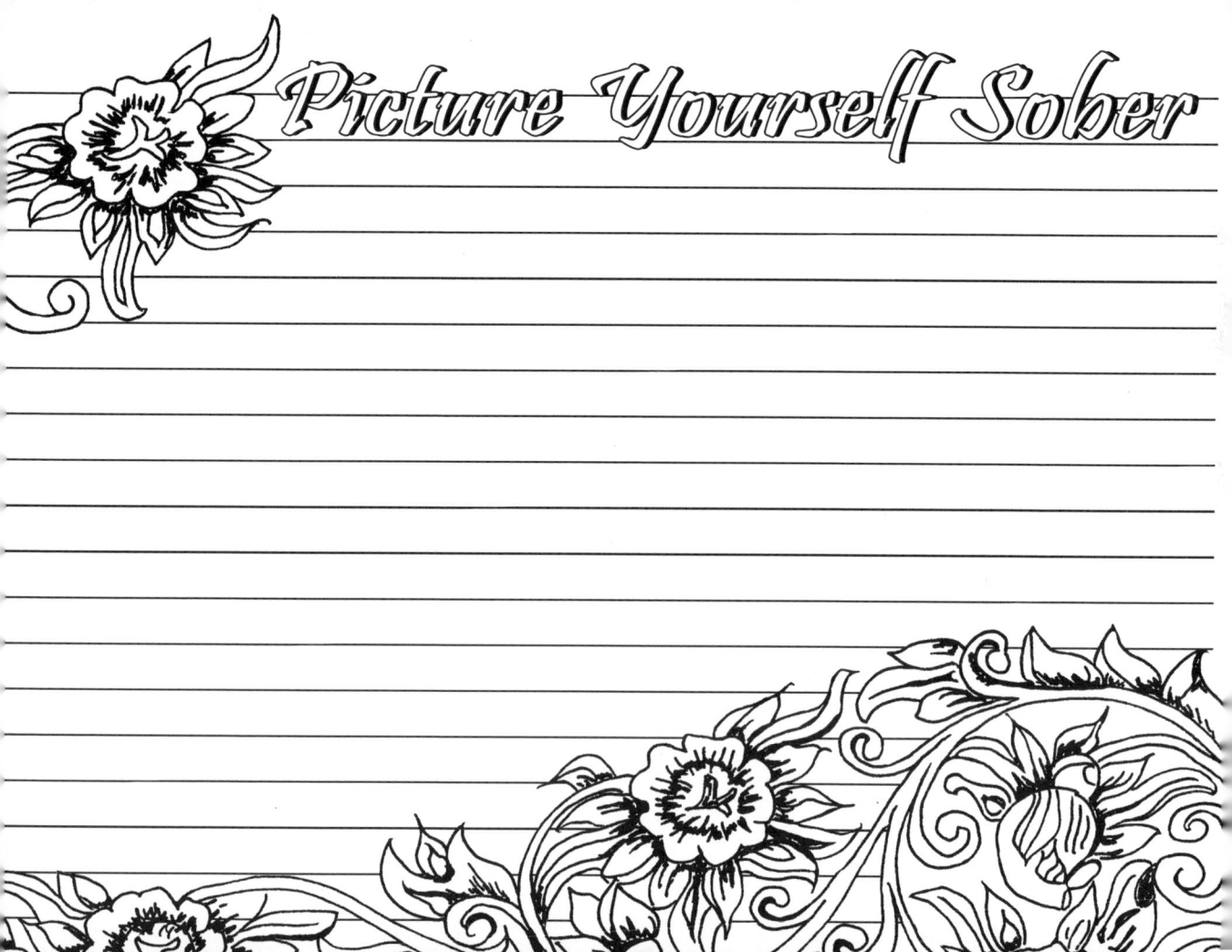

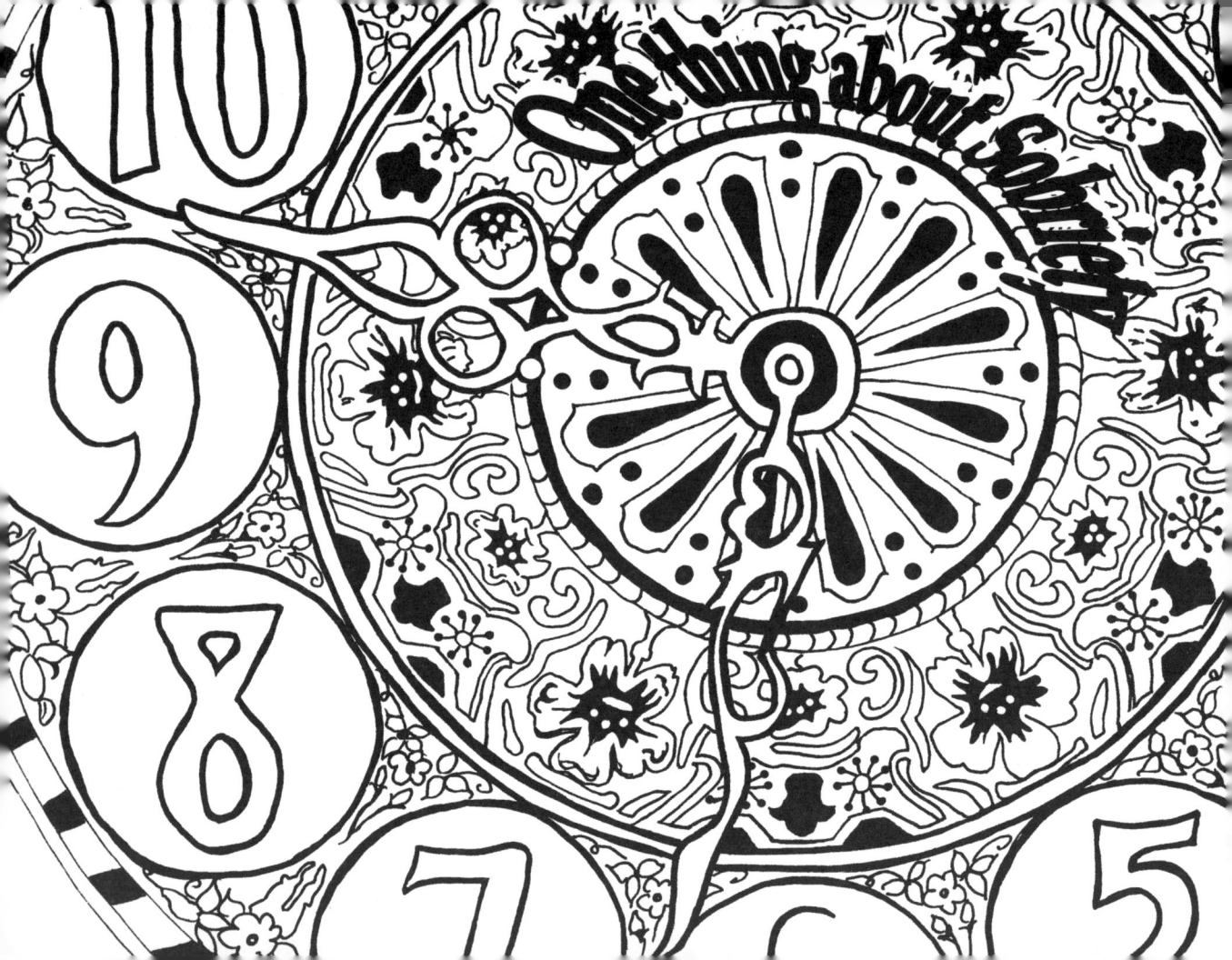

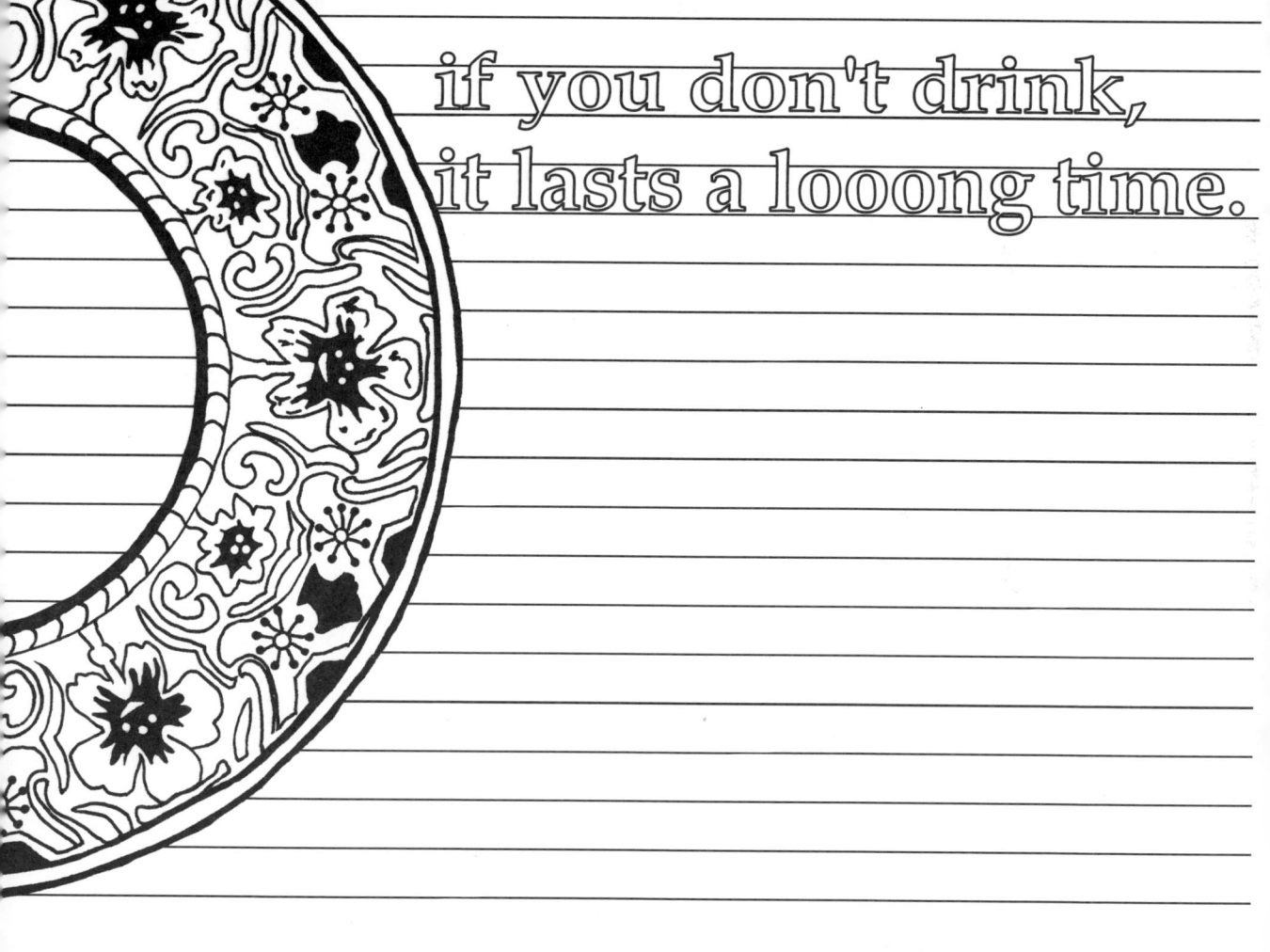

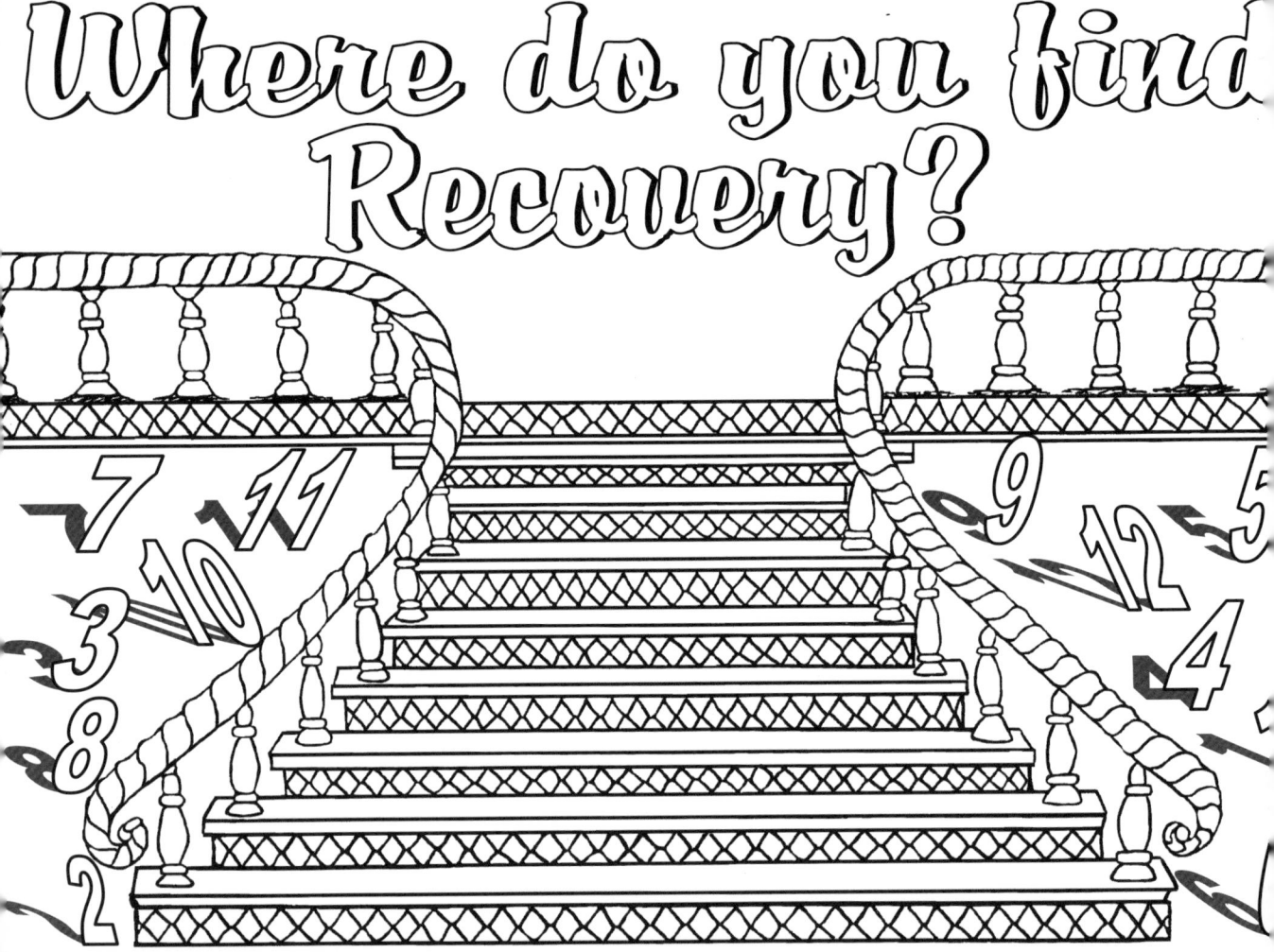

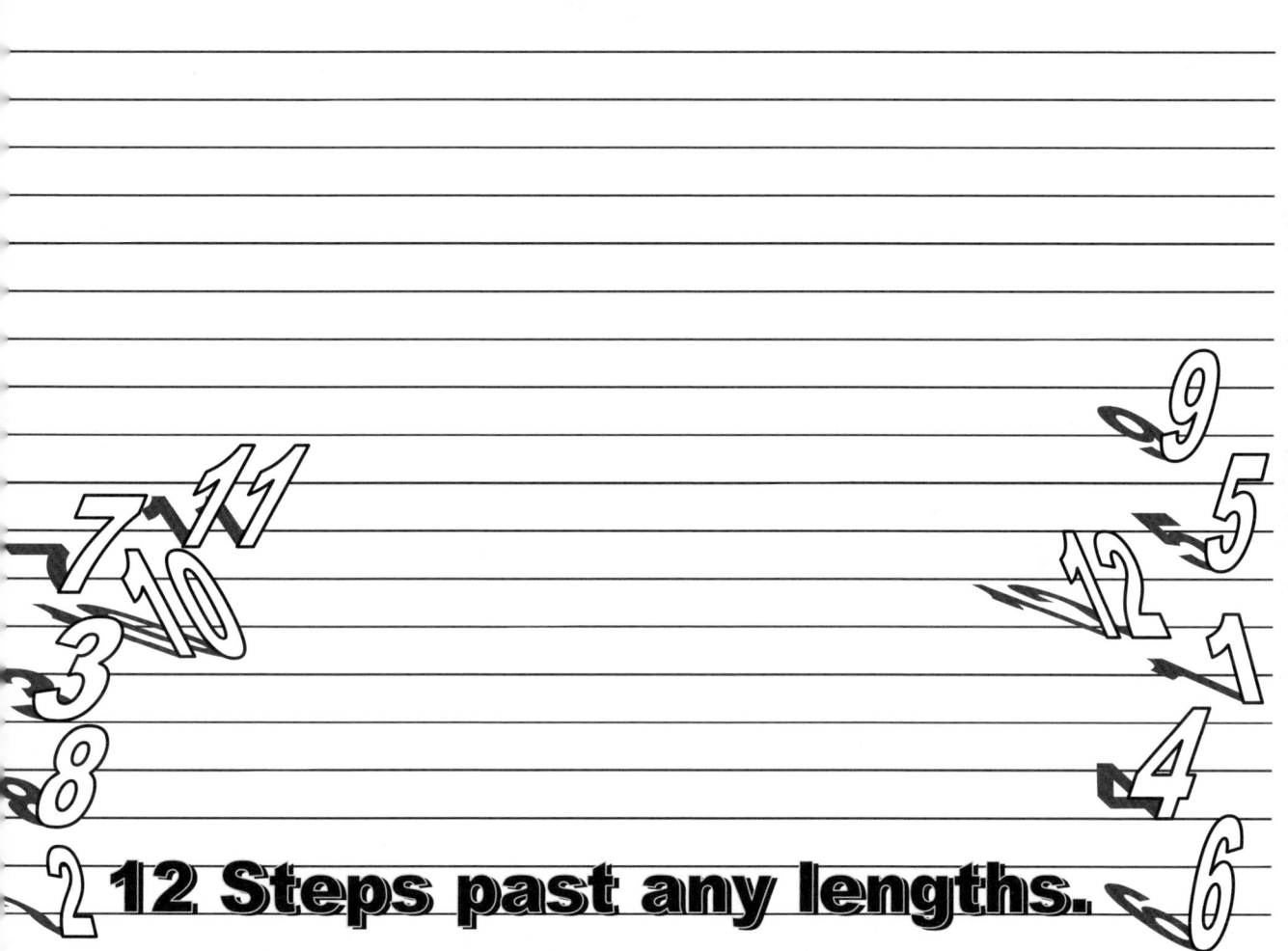

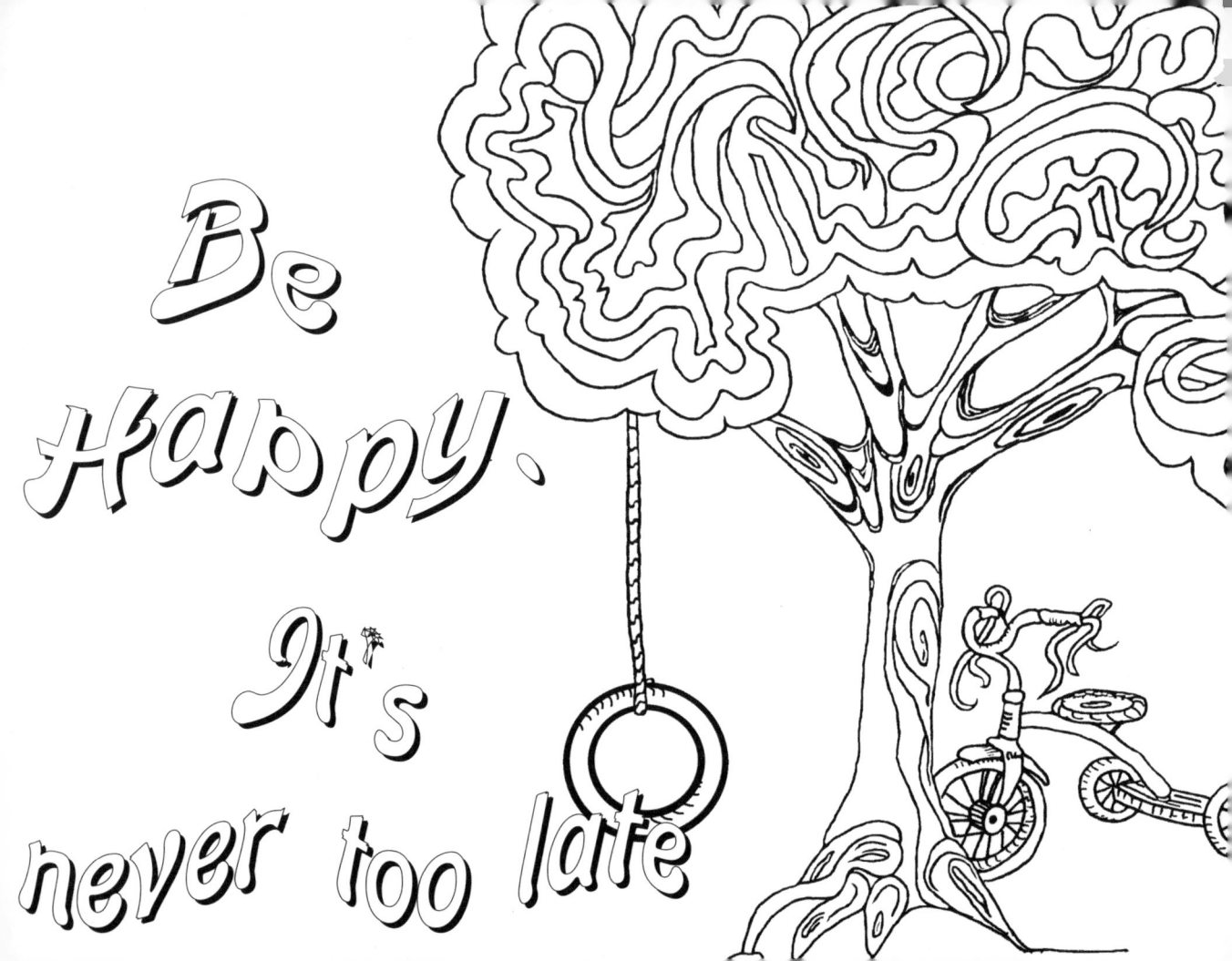

to have a happy childhood.

Be Happy
Be Happy
Be Be
Happy Happy

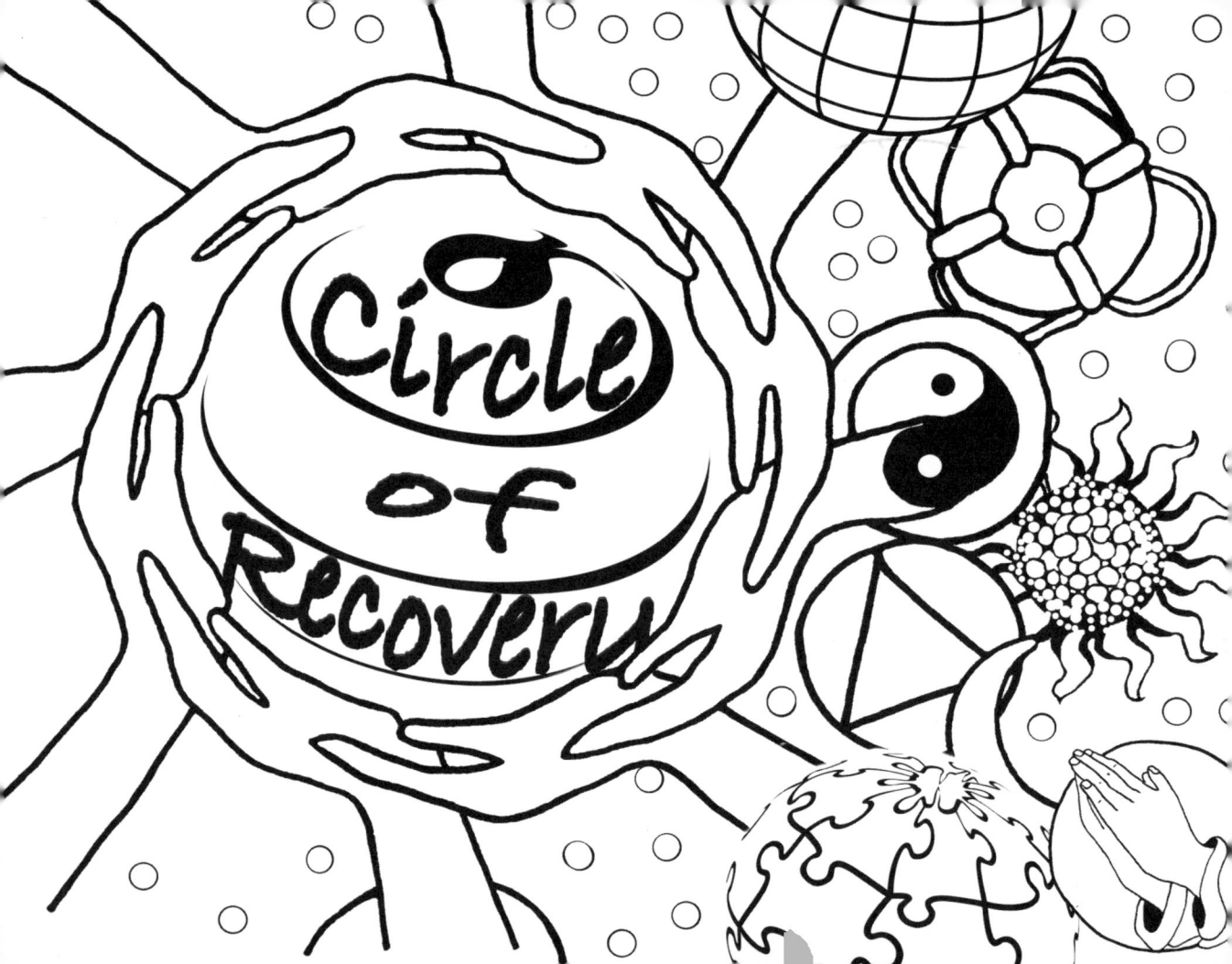

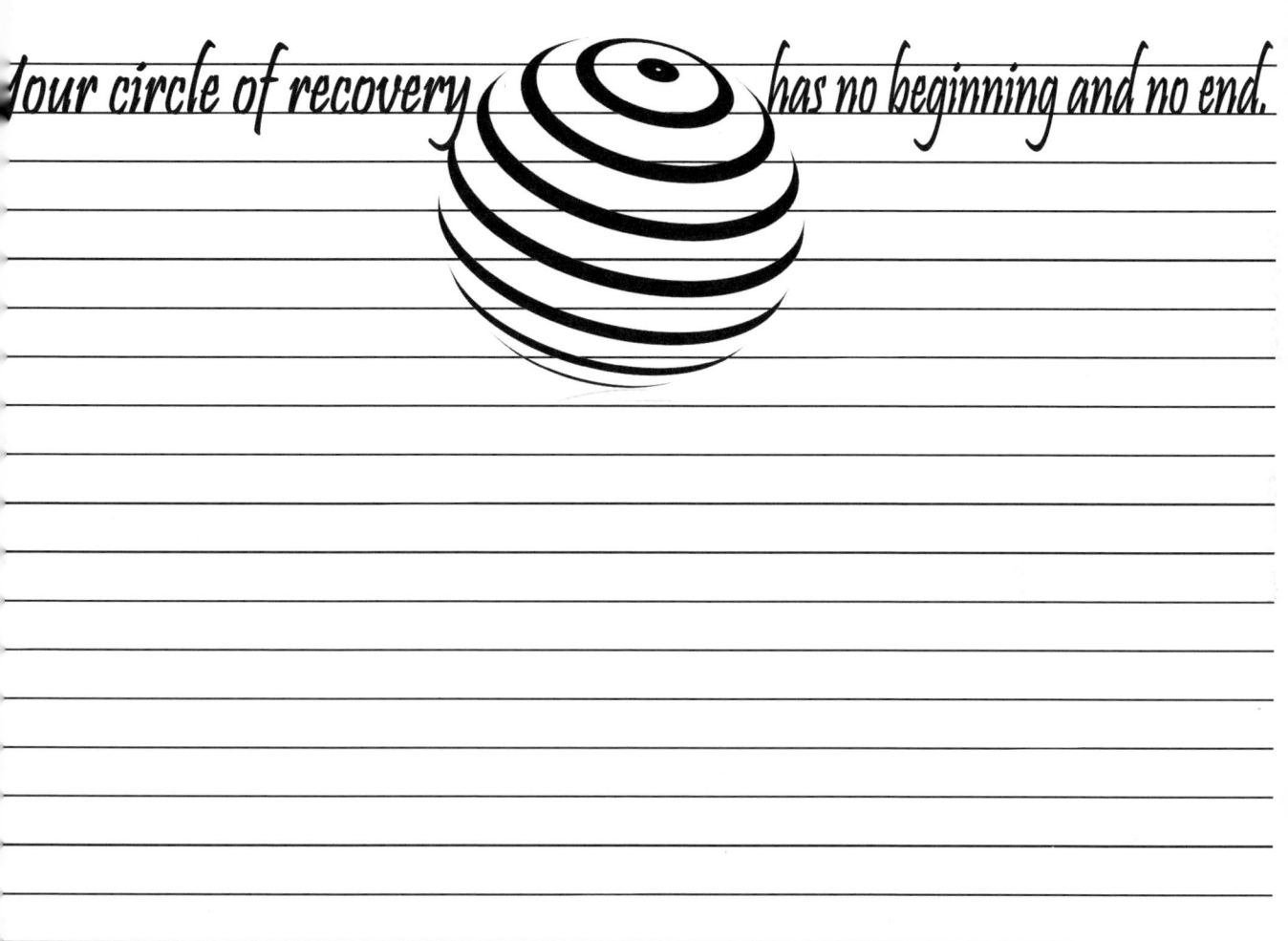

Your circle of recovery has no beginning and no end.

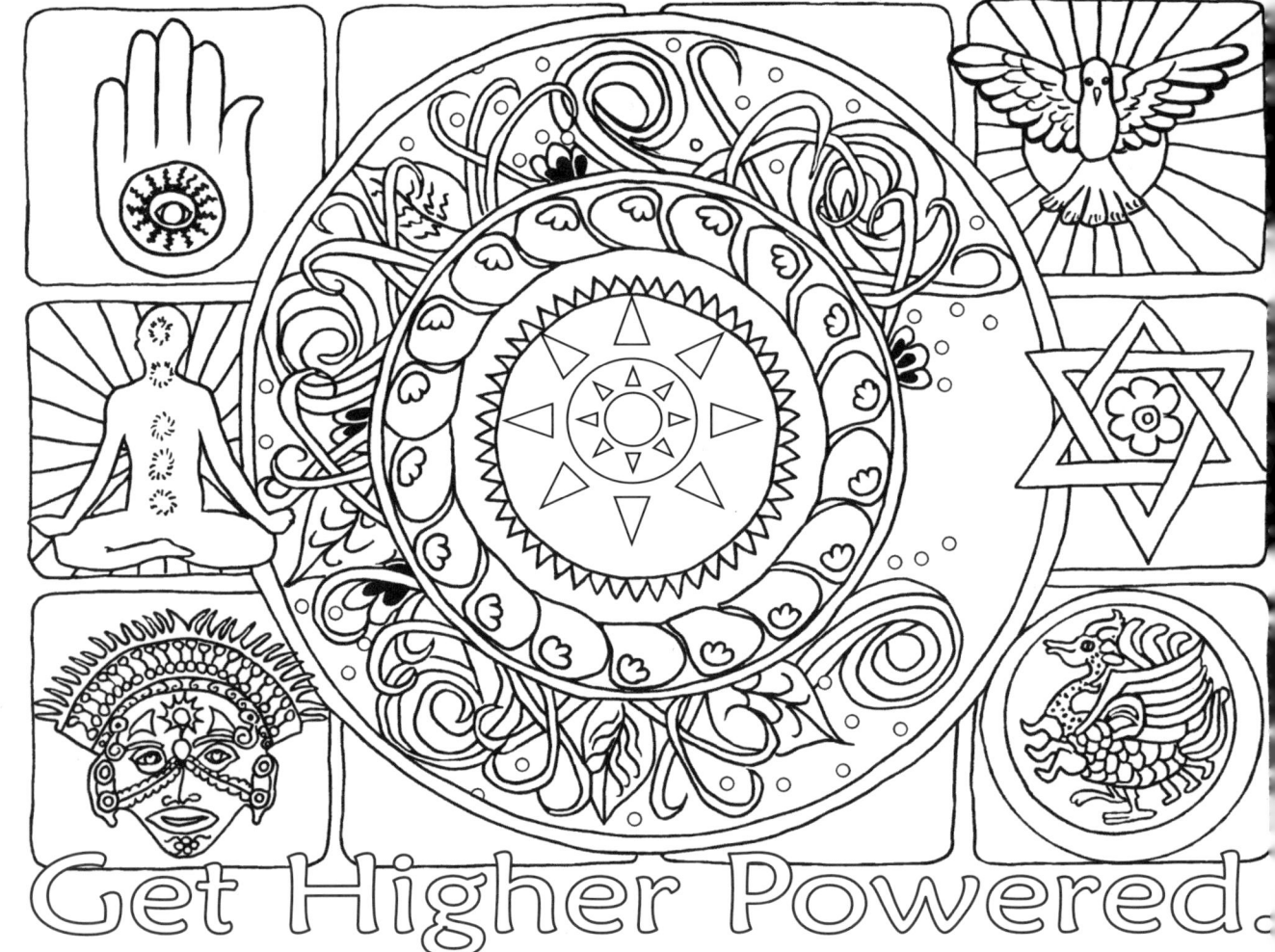

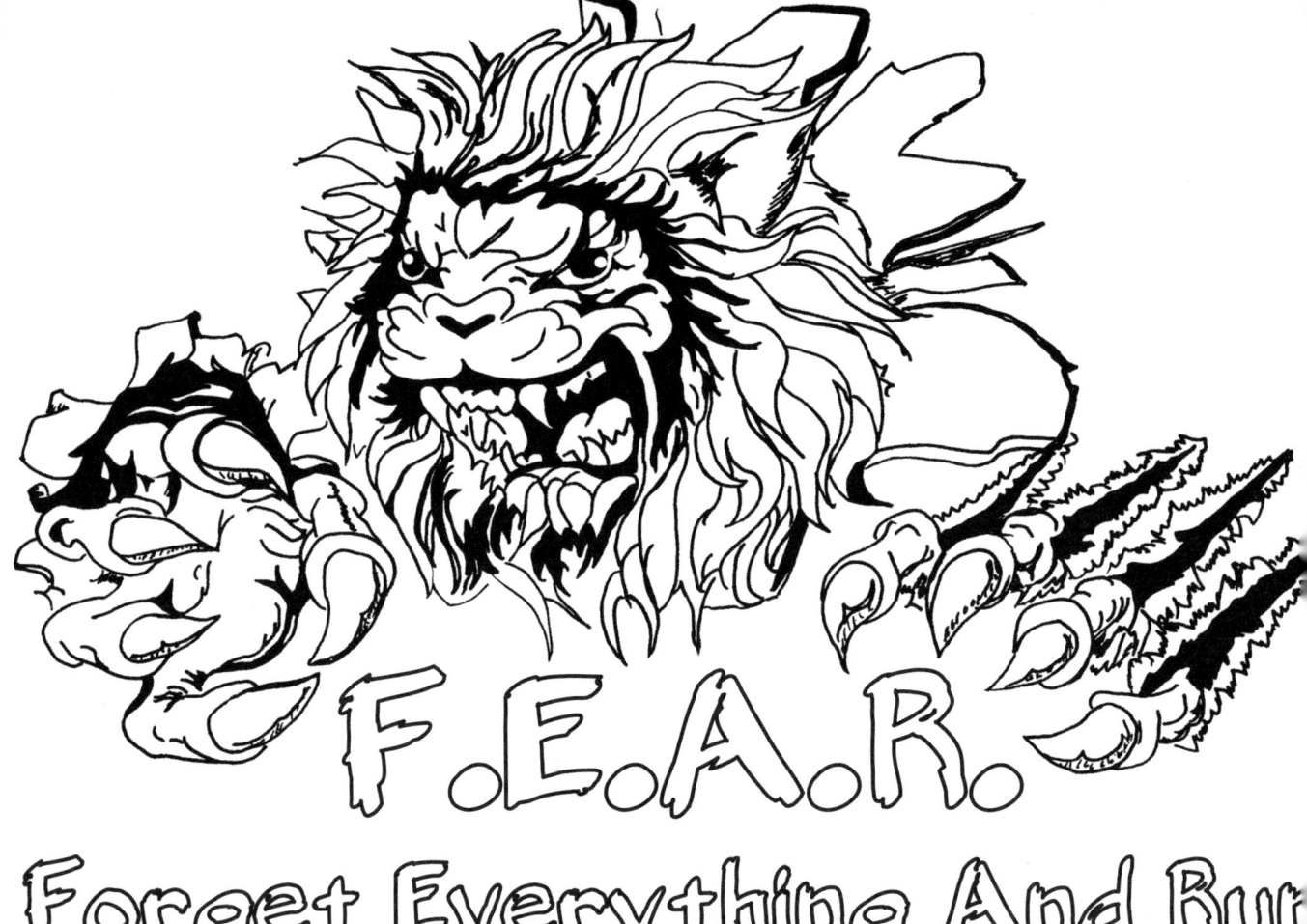

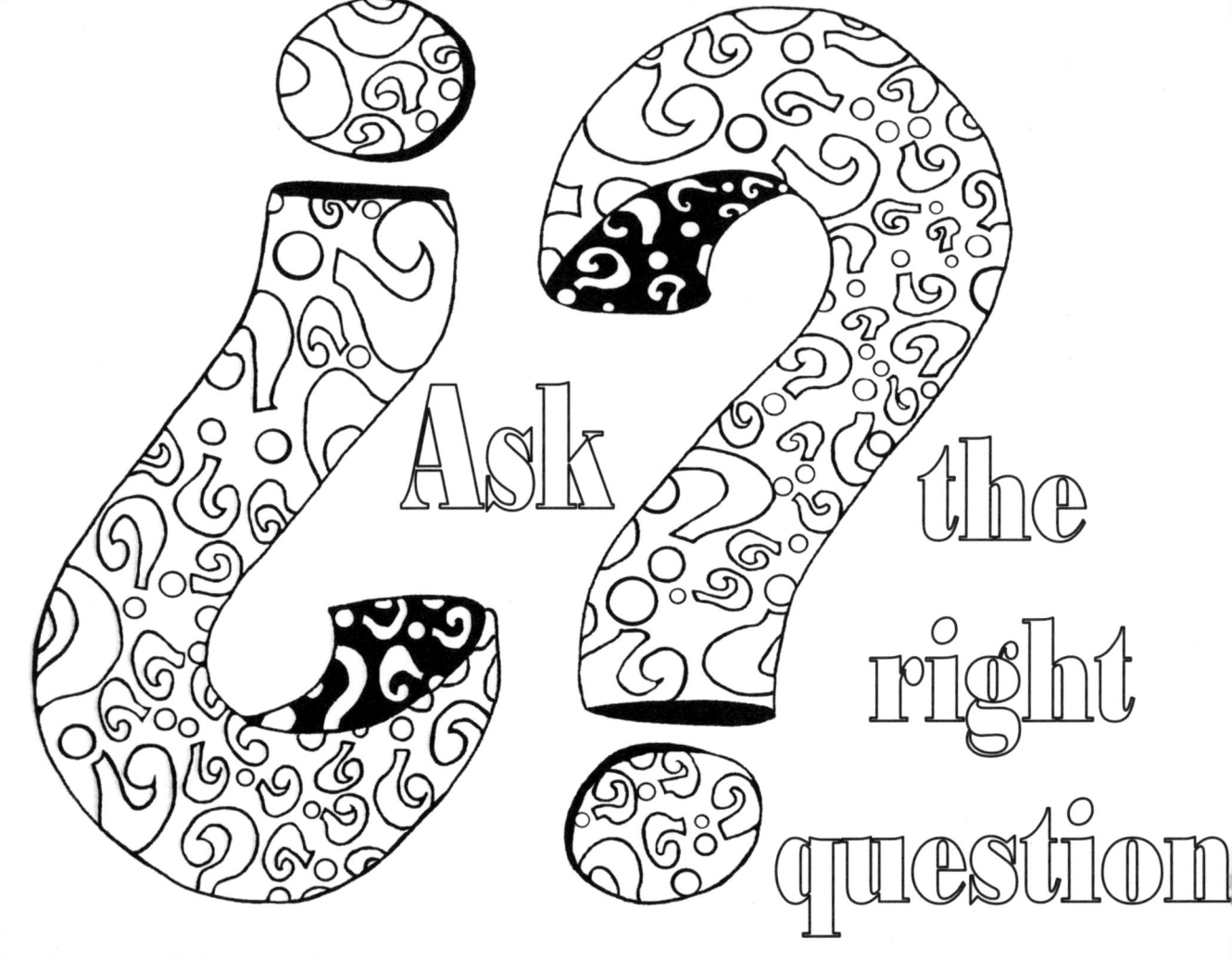

Get the right answer.

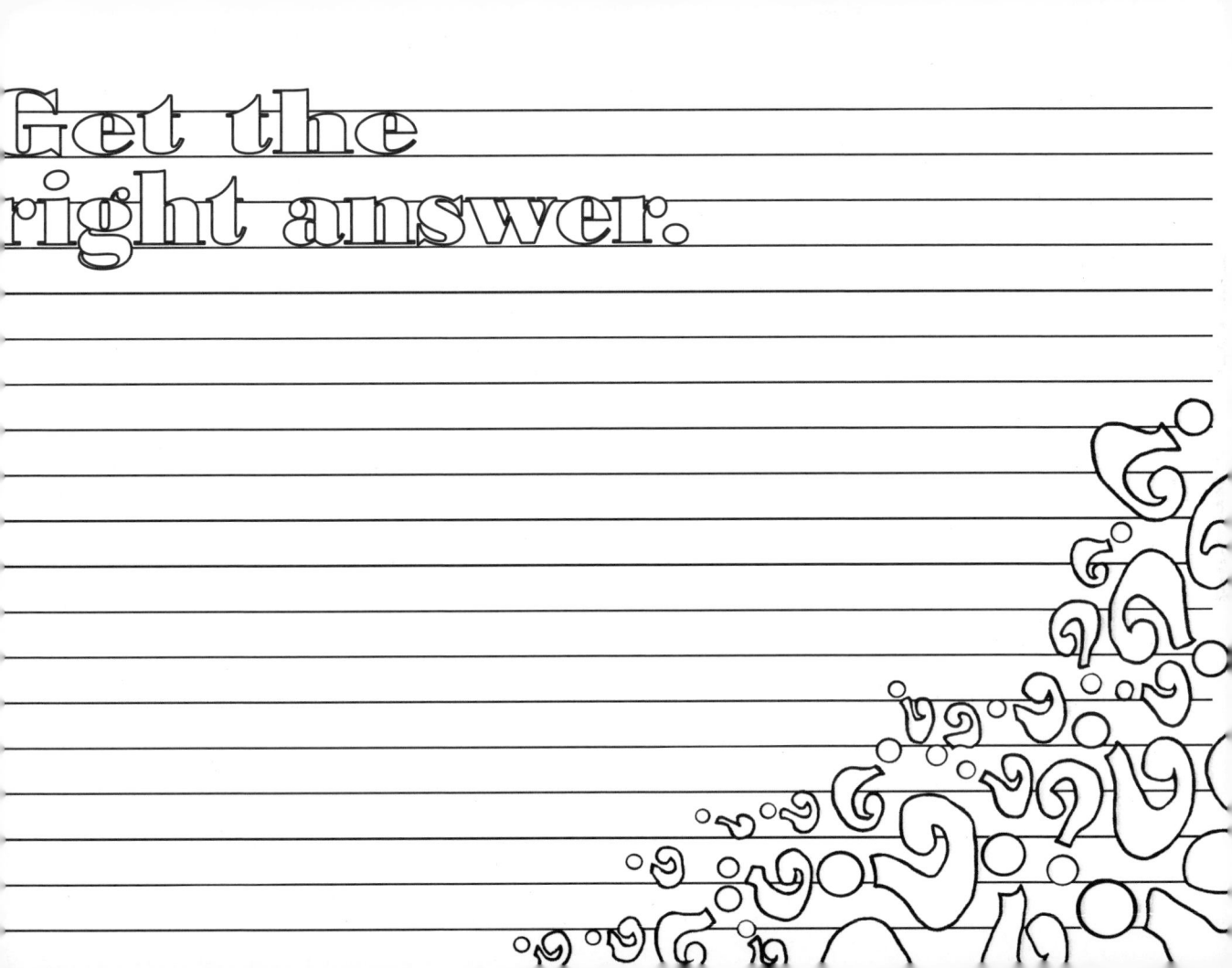

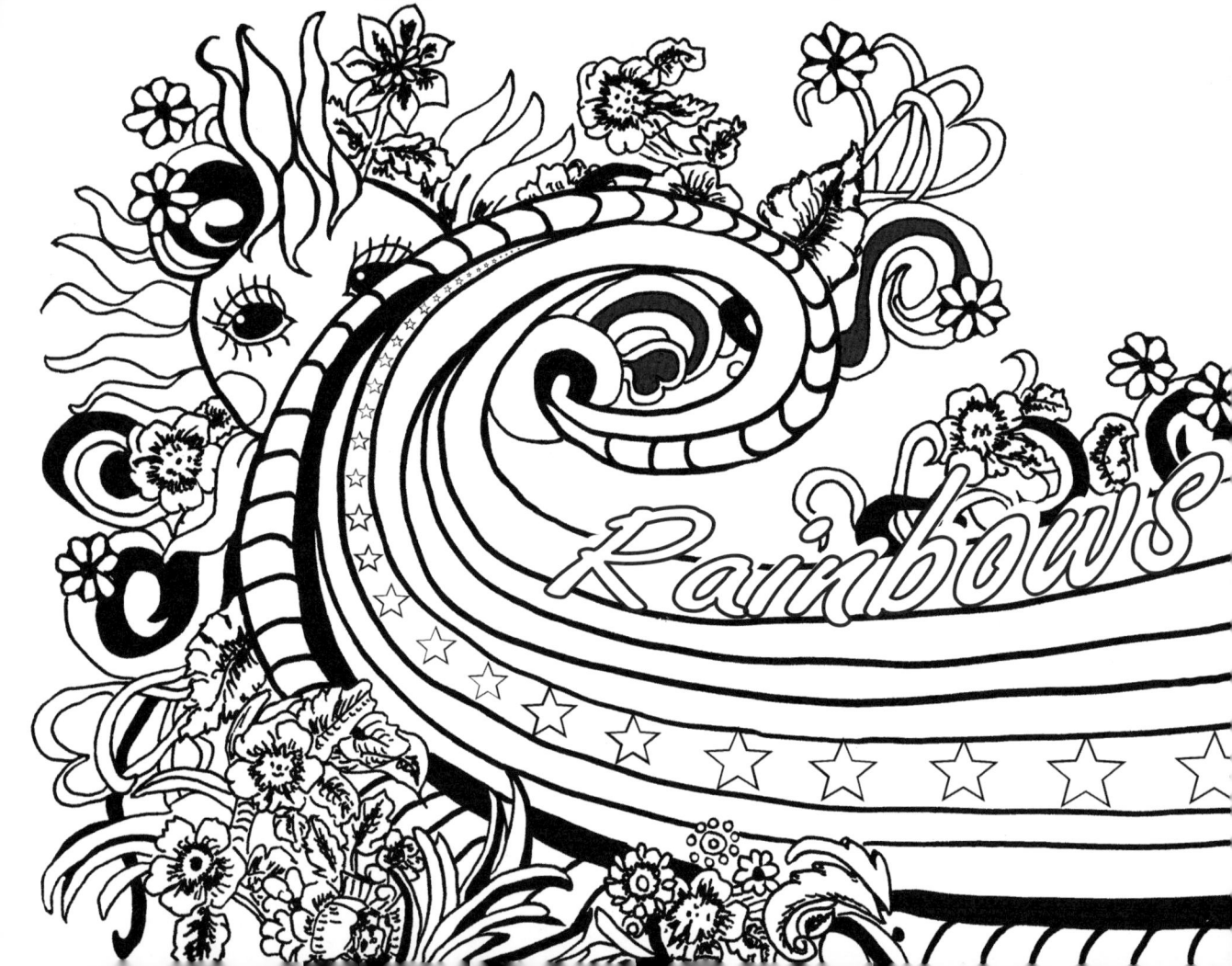

are the ribbons on God's gift to me,

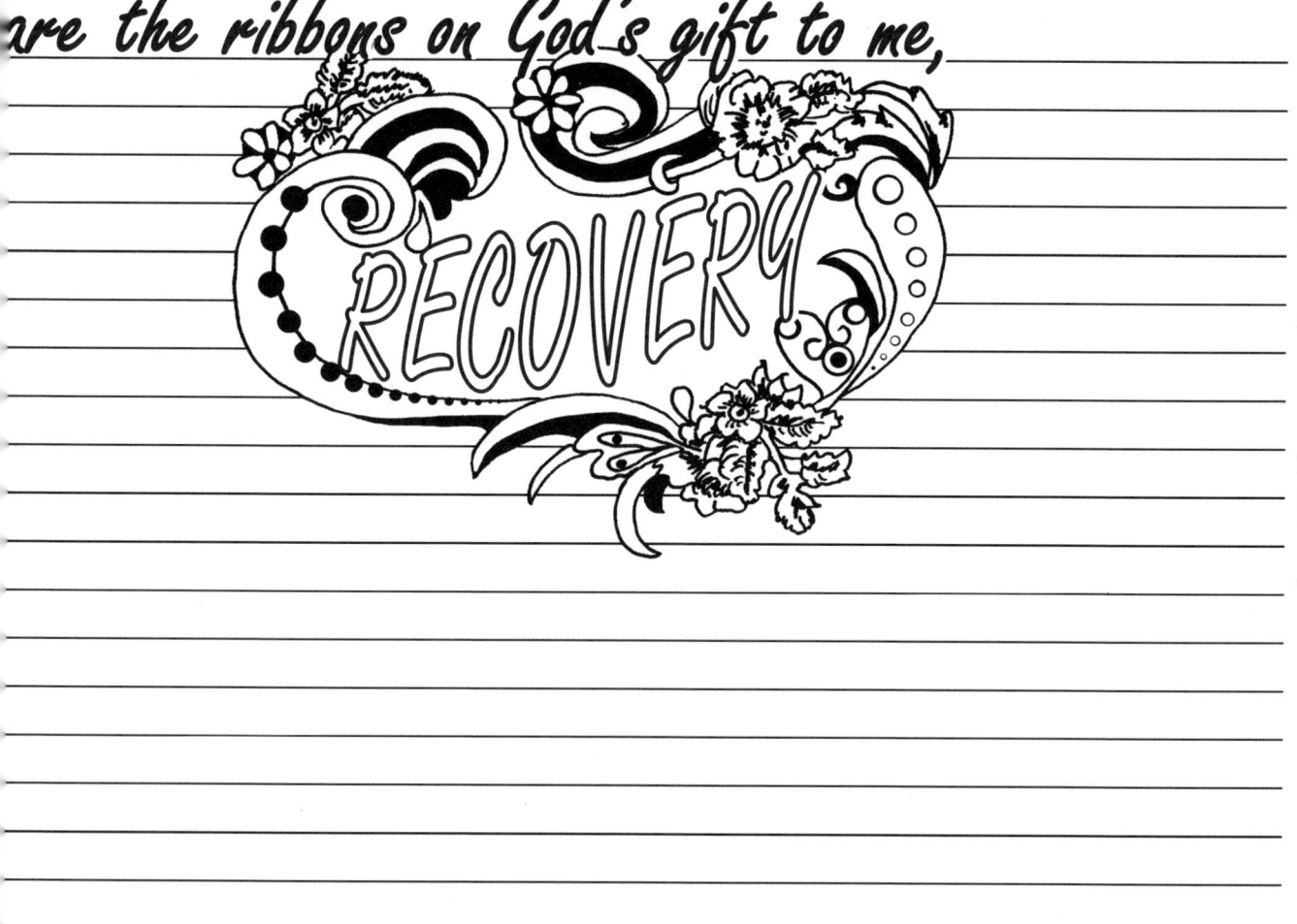

Day By Day Recovery Resources, Inc

Get Sober Like You Mean It

Day-By-Day.org

We don't publish a lot of titles but the ones we do, are the recovery books that people actually use. Written by and for those in recovery and inspired by the Old-timers, you won't find a better collection of 12 Step support anywhere.

DISCOUNTS

We offer up to 40% discount for groups and Institutions. For your next order please accept this **$10 Gift Certificate** toward any purchase at PocketSponsor.com/storefront.html (one time use) Write in "GIFT" at checkout.

In the meantime, please review some of our other great recovery books:

- PocketSponsor.com
- SittinginPictures.org
- YoungSoberFree.com
- 12StepDreamWork.com
- WalkSoftlyandCarryaBigBook.com
- RespectMeRules.com
- SoberCoachingYourTeen.com